Telephone Numbers and Information

Emergency Telephone Numbers

Emergency Medical Service (EMS): _____

Fire: _____

Police: _____

Poison Control Center: _____

Crisis Intervention Center: _____

Suicide Prevention Center: _____

Health Care Professionals

Physicians (internists, pediatricians, specialists):

Name	Specialty	Telephone Number
_____	_____	_____
_____	_____	_____
_____	_____	_____
_____	_____	_____

Dentist: _____

Employee Assistance Program (EAP): _____

Pharmacy: _____

24-Hour Pharmacy: _____

Hospital: _____

Health Insurance Information

Company: _____

Address: _____

Phone Number: _____

Policy Holder's Name: _____

Policy Number: _____

Social Security Number: _____

HealthySelf
The Guide to Self-Care and Wise Consumerism

Written by

Don R. Powell, Ph.D.

and the

American Institute for Preventive Medicine

Published by

American Institute for Preventive Medicine Press

Farmington Hills, Michigan

HealthySelf is one of a series of publications and programs offered by the American Institute for Preventive Medicine designed to help individuals reduce health care costs and improve the quality of their lives. Other booklets in the series include:

HealthyLife® Self-Care Guides - Each booklet addresses the most common health problems and teaches when to see the doctor or provide self care. Adult, Children's, Seniors', Women's, Spanish, Low Literacy and Emergency/First Aid editions are available.

All the Right Questions™ - guides individuals in making wise medical decisions.

Being a Wise Health Care Consumer™ - teaches people to be more knowledgeable about the health care system.

Healthy Savings™ - presents 101 tips on how to save money on medical care.

Toll-Free Hotlines to Health™ - allows your fingers to do the walking to over 150 health organizations that provide free advice, referrals and/or information.

Minding Your Mental Health™ - provides consumers with a guide to the mental health care field.

For more information, call or write:
American Institute for Preventive Medicine
30445 Northwestern Hwy., Suite 350
Farmington Hills, MI 48334
(810) 539-1800 / FAX (810) 539-1808

ACKNOWLEDGEMENTS:

The material in *HealthySelf* went through an extensive process in order to ensure medical accuracy and present the latest medical research. We are indebted to the physicians and other health professionals who served on our clinical review team.

Peter Fass, M.D., Medical Director, KeyCorp, Albany, NY

James Kohlenberg, M.D., Internal Medicine, John R Medical Clinic, Madison Heights, MI

Richard S. Lang, M.D., Head, Section of Occupational Medicine, Department of Preventive Medicine, Cleveland Clinic, Cleveland, OH

Dan Mayer, M.D., Associate Professor, Emergency Medicine, Albany Medical College, Director, Quality Improvement, Emergency Department, Albany Medical Center, Albany, NY

Susan Schooley, M.D., Chairman, Department of Family Practice, Henry Ford Health System, Detroit, MI

Charles B. Arnold, M.D., M.P.H., Medical Director, Medical Relations, Metropolitan Life Insurance Company, New York, NY

Jeffrey D. Band, M.D., Corporate Epidemiologist, Chief of Infectious Diseases and Medical Director, InterHealth: Health Care for International Travelers, William Beaumont Hospital, Royal Oak, MI

Ronald Berris, D.D.S., Team Dentist, Detroit Pistons basketball team and Family Dentistry, West Bloomfield, MI

Dwight L. Blackburn, M.D., Associate Medical Director, Blue Cross/Blue Shield of Kentucky, Louisville, KY

Dennis I. Blender, Ph.D., Psychologist, Plante Moran, Southfield, MI

Joyce Brownson-Booth, M.A., Director of Training, American Institute for Preventive Medicine, Dallas, TX

Marilyn Citron, M.S., M.A., Creative Consultant and Medical Writer, Birmingham, MI

Lynn DeGrande, A.C.S.W., CEAP, DeGrande & Associates, Senior Consultant, General Motors EAP, Detroit, MI

Frances B. DeHart, R.N., BSN, Director, Health Styles Corporate Health Risk Management, Greenville Hospital System, Greenville, SC

Kathy Foltner, M.A., CCA-A, Certified Audiologist, President, Audio-Vestibular Testing Center, Inc., Okemos, MI

Robin Foust, Director, Product and Marketing Development, Health Management Corporation, Richmond, VA

Elaine Frank, M.Ed., R.D., Vice President, American Institute for Preventive Medicine, Farmington Hills, MI

Barry A. Franklin, Ph.D., Director, Cardiac Rehabilitation and Exercise Laboratories, William Beaumont Hospital, Royal Oak, MI

Dwight D. Gaal, M.A., Director, Health Promotion, Bon Secours Hospital, Grosse Pointe, MI

Abe Gershonowicz, D.D.S., Family Dentistry, Sterling Heights, MI

Donald Hayes, M.D., Medical Director, Sara Lee Corporation, Winston-Salem, NC

William Hettler, M.D., Director, University Health Service, University of Wisconsin, Stevens Point, WI

Ronald Holmes, M.D., Co-Director, Division of General Pediatrics, Clinical Associate Professor of Pediatrics, Department of Pediatrics, University of Michigan Medical Center, Ann Arbor, MI

Susan Hoover, M.S., Director, Corporate/Community Services, Florida Hospital, Orlando, FL

Susan Horton, M.P.H., Director of Health Directors, Lexington Medical Center, West Columbia, SC

Jeanette Karwan, R.D., Director, Product Development, American Institute for Preventive Medicine, Farmington Hills, MI

Amy Kentera, M.P.H., Senior Vice President, Network Systems, Preferred Health Care, Wilton, CT

Ronald D. Kerwin, M.D., Clinical Instructor, Department of Dermatology, Wayne State University School of Medicine and Staff Physician, Crittenton Hospital, Rochester, MI and Sinai Hospital, Detroit, MI

Melvin Korobkin, M.D., Professor of Radiology, University of Michigan Medical School, Ann Arbor, MI

Martin Levinson, M.D., Chairman, Department of Pediatrics, Sinai Hospital, Detroit, MI

Acknowledgments, continued

Donald B. Levitt, Ph.D., Director, EAP, Owens Corning, Fiberglass, Toledo, OH

Herb Martin, Ph.D., Consultant, Enhanced Performance Systems, San Diego, CA

Tom Matlas, M.A., CEAP, CAC, Administrator, ReachOut EAP, Michigan Consolidated Gas Co., Detroit, MI

Richard N. Matzen, M.D., Emeritus Physician in Residence, The Cleveland Clinic Foundation, Cleveland, OH

James V. McConnell, Ph.D., Professor Emeritus of Psychology, University of Michigan, Ann Arbor, MI

Tony Mendes, Ph.D., Manager, Training and Development, AT&T Health Promotion, Basking Ridge, NJ

Michael P. O'Donnell, M.P.H., M.B.A., Publisher, American Journal of Health Promotion, Rochester Hills, MI

Thomas C. Overhold, M.D., Department of Internal Medicine and Pediatrics, Henry Ford Hospital, Detroit, MI

Philip Parker, M.D., Clinical Assistant Professor, Department of Psychiatry, Wayne State University School of Medicine; Psychiatrist, Private Practice, Southfield, MI

Owen Z. Perlman, M.D., Director, Department of Physical Medicine and Rehabilitation, Catherine McAuley Health Center, Ann Arbor, MI

William H. Rattner, M.D., Adjunct Assistant Professor, Department of Urology, Wayne State University School of Medicine and Staff Physician, Sinai Hospital, Detroit, MI

Edward J. Roccella, Ph.D., M.P.H., Coordinator, National High Blood Pressure Education Program, Office of Preventive Education and Control, National Heart, Lung and Blood Institute, Bethesda, MD

F. David Rollo, M.D., Ph.D., President and CEO, MetriCor, Louisville, KY

Michael Rontal, M.D., F.A.C.S., Clinical Assistant Professor, University of Michigan Medical School and Wayne State University School of Medicine and Staff Physician, Sinai Hospital, Detroit, MI and William Beaumont Hospital, Royal Oak, MI

Susan Herman Ryskamp, M.S., R.D., Training Coordinator, American Institute for Preventive Medicine, Farmington Hills, MI

E.A. Shaptini, M.D., Vice President and Medical Director, American Natural Resources Company, Detroit, MI

William Solomon, M.D., Clinical Instructor, Department of Internal Medicine, Wayne State University School of Medicine and Medical Director, Jewish Home for the Aged, Detroit, MI

Steven Starr, D.P.M., Director, Birmingham Foot Care, Birmingham, MI

Neill D. Varner, D.O., M.P.H., Medical Director, Saginaw Steering Division, General Motors Corporation, Saginaw, MI, member of the UAW-GM Health Promotion Task Force and Medical Director, Saginaw County Department of Public Health

Marvin S. Weckstein, M.D., Psychotherapy and Outpatient Psychiatry, Assistant Director of Adult Psychiatry Training, Fairlawn Center, Pontiac, MI

Mark Werner, M.D. Obstetrics and Gynecology, Staff Physician, William Beaumont Hospital, Royal Oak, MI

Yael Zoldan, Manager, Graphic Design, American Institute for Preventive Medicine, Farmington Hills, MI

We would also like to thank the following persons from Lewis Gale, Clinic, Salem, VA

Douglas D. Blevins, M.D., Infectious Disease, Internal Medicine

Gary P. Gross, M.D., Dermatologist

J. Bruce Hagadorn, M.D., Otolarygologist

William J. Kagey, M.D., Pediatrician

Julie T. Lusk, M.Ed., Director of Health Management

Alonzo H. Myers, Jr., M.D., Orthopaedic Surgeon

Joseph L. Nelson, III, M.D., Gastroenterologist

E. Blackford Noland, M.D., Internal Medicine

Mark A. Schmidt, M.D., Urologist

Bruce Stewart, M.D., Internal Medicine

J. Steven Strosnider, M.D., Director of Psychological Counseling

David J. Thaler, D.O., Internal Medicine

Table of Contents

SECTION I
Wise Medical Consumerism

Introduction

Section I helps you learn to be a wise medical consumer. Chapters 1 through 6 give many tips and guidelines to help you use the health care system wisely. Chapter 7 offers information on what you should do about basic dental health. Chapter 8 lists common mental health problems and reasons to seek help for them. Ways to stay well and prevent disease are presented in Chapter 9. This section combines important information and a common sense approach to make it easier for you and your family to take responsibility for your own health and well-being.

chapter ❶
YOU & YOUR DOCTOR

Choosing a Doctor

Selecting a doctor takes great care. The guidelines below can help.

- ▭ Find out if the doctor accepts your health insurance. If you belong to a Health Maintenance Organization (HMO), you will need to go to participating doctors. You may be able to choose among many doctors within the plan.
- ▭ Ask relatives and friends for recommendations. A "good reputation" means a lot.
- ▭ Check with the local medical society. You can specify what type of doctor, you are looking for by location, gender, specialty and age.
- ▭ Look for a doctor whom you can relate to and meets your expectations of how medical decisions are made. (The doctor alone, you alone, you and the doctor together).
- ▭ Call the American Board of Medical Specialists (ABMS) at 1-800-776-2378 to find out if the doctor is "Board Certified" or "Board Eligible," and the board or boards under which the physician has received certification. "Board Certified" means that he/she has two or more years of training in a specialty after graduation from medical school and has passed a national examination. "Board Eligible" means that the training has been completed, but not the exam. The local medical society can provide this information, but remember, these credentials do not guarantee that a doctor is competent.

- ▭ Interview several doctors before you decide on the one you want. Find out if you agree on general health philosophies and treatment approaches.
- ▭ Ask about office hours, staffing, fees, and if the doctor makes house calls. Find out how long you must wait for an appointment.
- ▭ Ask about the office policy regarding payment. Ask whether you must pay for your visit at that time or whether you can be billed and pay later.
- ▭ Find out if the doctor is alone or in a group practice. If alone, ask what other doctors serve as back-ups.
- ▭ Find out which hospital the doctor sends patients to and if your health insurance is accepted there.

Finding the right doctor for you is a big part of being a wise medical consumer. Look for a doctor who:

- ▭ Is competent and can care for all your general health needs, or can refer you to other appropriate health care providers for any special health needs.
- ▭ You feel comfortable with.
- ▭ You trust.

Doctors and Their Specialties

The most common specialists and what they do are:

Allergist - Diagnoses and treats allergies.

Anesthesiologist - Administers anesthetics that are used during surgery.

Cardiologist - Diagnoses and treats diseases of the heart and blood vessels.

Dermatologist - Diagnoses and treats diseases and problems of the skin.

Emergency Medicine - Specializes in rapid recognition and treatment of trauma or acute illness.

Endocrinologist - Diagnoses disorders of the internal glands, such as the thyroid and adrenal glands.

Family Practitioner - Provides total health care of the individual and the family. Scope is not limited by age, gender or organ system.

Gastroenterologist - Diagnoses and treats disorders of the digestive tract: stomach, bowels, liver, gallbladder and related organs.

Gynecologist - Diagnoses and treats disorders of the female reproductive system.

Internist - Diagnoses and treats diseases, especially those of adults.

Nephrologist - Diagnoses and treats diseases and problems of the kidneys.

Neurologist - Diagnoses and treats disorders of the nervous system.

Obstetrician - Provides care and treatment of females during pregnancy, labor and delivery, and six weeks after delivery.

Oncologist - Diagnoses and treats all types of cancer and other types of benign and malignant tumors.

Ophthalmologist - Diagnoses, monitors and treats vision problems and other disorders of the eye, and prescribes prescription lenses.

Orthopedist - Diagnoses and treats skeletal injuries and diseases of the bones and muscles.

Otolaryngologist - Diagnoses and treats disorders that affect the ears, respiratory and upper alimentary systems (in general, the head and neck).

Pathologist - Examines and diagnoses organs, tissues and body fluids.

Pediatrician - Diagnoses and treats the physical, emotional and social problems of children.

Physiatrist - Provides physical and rehabilitative treatment of muscle and bone disorders.

Psychiatrist - Treats and prevents mental, emotional and/or behavioral disorders.

Radiologist - Uses X-rays and radiant energy for diagnosis and treatment of disease.

Urologist - Diagnoses and treats diseases of the urinary or urogential tract.

Calling Your Doctor Checklist

There will be times when you must call your doctor or other health care provider. Find these things out in advance:

- ▭ What is the best time to call?
- ▭ What is the doctor's rule for returning calls?
- ▭ Who should you speak with (i.e., physician's assistant, nurse, etc.) if the doctor can't come to the phone?
- ▭ What is the phone number for emergency calls or calls when the office is closed?
- ▭ Who can you call if your doctor is out of town?

When you reach your doctor or other health care provider by phone, be prepared to:

- ▭ Get to the point of your call quickly, especially if you've phoned after hours. (Have someone else call the doctor for you if you are unable to talk).
- ▭ Define your problems and symptoms. Write these down and keep them by the telephone so you can report them quickly and completely.
- ▭ Report results of self tests and things you have been keeping track of, such as temperature of 101°F degrees for two days, diarrhea that has lasted for 48 hours, etc.
- ▭ Ask the doctor what you should do. Write it down.
- ▭ Have your pharmacist's phone number handy in case the doctor needs to prescribe medicine.
- ▭ Ask if and when you should call back, or if you should come to the office.
- ▭ Ask what things might occur which would require you to go to the emergency room.
- ▭ Thank the doctor for talking to you on the telephone.

Making the Most of a Doctor Visit

Patients often feel rushed or uneasy at the doctor's office. And when you're sick, there is a tendency to feel vulnerable and passive. Plan ahead of time what you want to discuss with the doctor. Write it down and take it with you. Be prepared to talk about your current problems and symptoms and needs. Also be able to state your medical history.

What Your Doctor Should Know about You

Aside from a general health history, it is important that your doctor know about the following:

Dietary habits - Are you a frequent junk-food eater? Are you especially fond of cheesecake, sour cream, or other fatty foods?

Your occupation - Do you work in a high-stress job? Are you exposed to nickel, nuclear power radiation, or other toxic substances?

Sleep habits - Do you frequently awaken before dawn or have problems getting to sleep?

Family problems - Are you currently going through a divorce?

Lifestyle - Do you get any exercise?

Stress - Do you work in a noisy environment?

Health attitude - Are you serious about quitting smoking, getting more exercise or eating better?

History of family illness - Does heart disease, high blood pressure, diabetes, kidney problems, or cancer run in your family?

Major life events - Have you recently retired from work, gotten married or had a child?

Living arrangements - Do you live alone?

Doctor-Patient Communication

Communication is a two-way process. Listening as well as speaking to one another is something both doctor and patient must work on together. Being honest and open with each other is also important. The more honest you are, the better your doctor can help you. You can make the most of your doctor-patient communication with these suggestions:

- Plan what you will say to your doctor about your problem ahead of time. Your observations about a health problem can be invaluable in making a diagnosis.
- Repeat in your own words what the doctor has told you. Use simple phrases like, "Do I hear you say that . . . ?" or "My understanding of the problem is . . . "
- Take notes on what is wrong and what you need to do.
- If you are confused by medical terms, ask for simple definitions. There is no need to be embarrassed by this. When a medication is prescribed, ask about its possible side effects, its effectiveness, and how long it must be taken. If your doctor discusses surgery, ask about alternatives, risks, and a second opinion.
- Be frank with the doctor if any part of the office visit is annoying, such as lengthy waiting time or discourteous staff. Be tactful, but honest.
- Don't be afraid to voice your fears about what you've heard. The doctor may be able to clarify any misconceptions.
- Discuss anything you've done that has relieved symptoms or that has made them worse.
- Find out the best time to call your doctor if you have any questions after you leave the office.

Rating Your Doctor

In order to feel good about your medical care, you should feel good about your doctor, too. Ask yourself the following questions to evaluate your physician.

- Does your doctor listen to you and answer all your questions about the causes and treatment of your medical problems, or is he or she vague, impatient, or unwilling to answer?
- Are you comfortable with your doctor? Can you openly discuss your feelings and talk about personal concerns, including sexual and emotional problems?
- Does your doctor take a thorough history, asking about past physical and emotional problems, family medical history, medications you are taking, and other matters affecting your health?
- Does your doctor address the root causes of your medical problems or simply prescribe medications to treat the symptoms?
- Are you satisfied with the doctor's substitute when he or she is unavailable?
- Do you feel at ease asking your doctor questions that may sound "silly"?
- Does your doctor explain things in simple terms?
- Is the office staff friendly? Do they listen to you?
- Does your doctor answer your telephone calls promptly?
- Are you generally kept waiting for a long time when you have an appointment?
- Does the doctor have hospital privileges at a respected hospital?

If you are not satisfied with your answers to these questions, discuss your concerns with your doctor. If, after this discussion, you are still not satisfied, consider looking for another doctor.

chapter 2

MEDICAL EXAMS & TESTS

Having a Routine Checkup

The routine physical exam from a doctor or at a health clinic is a way to find out about the state of your health. It also allows you to ask your doctor questions and to benefit from finding out if you have a health problem you don't know about. Some diseases like high blood pressure and some cancers may not have any symptoms in the early stages. Tests your doctor does can help detect these. Check the chart on page 17 for when health tests and check ups are recommended.

The basic parts of a check-up are:
- A complete medical history (questions on family health history, previous illness, emotional well-being).
- A check on how well body organs are functioning (eyes, ears, heart, skin, bowels, etc.).
- Checking the vital signs (blood pressure, pulse, breathing rate, temperature).
- Actual body examination (listening, thumping and looking at specific body parts).
- Routine diagnostic tests (blood tests, X-rays, etc.).
- A check of specific health concerns.

Tests and What They are For

Blood Pressure Test - Checks two kinds of pressure within the blood vessels. The higher number (systolic blood pressure) gauges the pressure when your heart is pumping and the lower number (diastolic blood pressure) represents the pressure between heartbeats. High blood pressure is a symptomless disease that can lead to a heart attack and/or a stroke.

Vision - Checks for marked changes or degeneration of eye functioning.

Pap Smear - Is used to detect the early signs of cervical cancer, uterine cancer and herpes.

Mammography - An X-ray to detect breast tumors or problems.

Professional Breast Exam - A physician or nurse examines the breasts for signs of abnormalities.

Digital Rectal Exam - Checks for early signs of colorectal and/or prostate abnormalities including cancer.

Stool Blood Test - Checks for early signs of colorectal abnormalities including cancer.

Sigmoidoscopy - Checks for early signs of colorectal abnormalities and cancer.

Cholesterol Blood Test - Checks the levels of fatty deposits (cholesterol) in the blood. High cholesterol levels are linked to heart disease.

Glaucoma Screening - Checks for increased pressure within the eye. Glaucoma can result in blindness if not treated.

Common Health Tests
& How Often to Have Them

AGES		20-29	30-39	40-49	50 and older
Physical Exam		Every 2-3 years	Every 2-3 years	Every 2-3 years	Every 1-2 years
Blood Pressure		Every 1-2 years	Every 1-2 years	Every 1-2 years	Every 1-2 years
Vision		Every 3-5 years	Every 3-5 years	Every 3-5 years	Every 2-3 years
Pap Test[1]	W	Every 2-3 years	Every 2-3 years	Every 2-3 years	Every year
Mammography[2]	O				Every year
Breast Self-Examination*	M E	Monthly	Monthly	Monthly	Monthly
Professional Breast Examination	N			Every year	Every year
Testicular Self-Exam (Men)**		Discuss With Your Doctor			
Digital Rectal Exam				Discuss With Your Doctor	
Stool Blood Test					Every year
Sigmoidoscopy					Every 3-5 years
Cholesterol Blood Test[3]		Every 3-5 years	Every 3-5 years	Every 3-5 years	Every 3-5 years
Glaucoma Screening[4]					Every 2-3 years
Regular Dental Checkup		Every year	Every year	Every year	Every year

Legend:
- ■ Every year
- ▯ Every 1-2 years
- ▨ Every 2-3 years
- ▧ Every 3-5 years

Note: Recommendations for routine medical exams may vary. These apply only to healthy people who do not have symptoms of illnesses. If you have an increased risk of a particular illness, testing may need to be done sooner or more often. Extra tests may also need to be done. Follow your doctor's advice. Also, check with your insurance company to see if and when tests are covered.

1. Pap tests should start at age 18 or under age 18 if sexual activity has begun. They should be given every year until tests are normal 3 years in a row. Thereafter, pap tests should be given at least every three years. *[Note: The American College of Obstetricians and Gynecologists recommends an annual pap test.]*
2. As recommended by The National Cancer Institute. Check with your doctor for his or her recommendations.
3. The National Cholesterol Education Program (NCEP) recommends a blood cholesterol test at least once every 5 years, and that high-density lipoprotein (HDL) be part of initial cholesterol testing.
4. Glaucoma screening is recommended earlier for African Americans. It should be done every 2 to 3 years between the ages 40 and 49.

* See pages 137 and 138 for a step-by-step breast self-examination guide.
** See page 149 for how to do a testicular self-exam.

Immunization Schedule

	Immunizations						When & Where		
Age	Hepatitis B (HB)[1]	Oral Polio (OPV)	Diphtheria Tetanus Pertussis (DTP)	H. influenzae type b (Hib)[3]	Measles Mumps Rubella (MMR)[4]	Varicella Zoster Virus Vaccine (VZV)[5]	Name	Name	
Birth	HB Birth - 2 mos.								
2 mos.	HB 2-4 mos.	OPV	DTP	Hib					
4 mos.		OPV	DTP	Hib					
6 mos.	HB 6-18 mos.	OPV 6-18 mos.	DTP	Hib					
12-15 mos.			DTP 12-18 mos.	Hib	MMR	VZV 12-18 mos.			
4-6 years		OPV	DTP		MMR[4]				
11-16 years			T(d)[2] and every 10 years thereafter						

Recommendations through age 16 were approved by the Advisory Committee on Immunization Practice (ACIP), the American Academy of Pediatrics (AAP), and the American Academy of Family Physicians (AAFP), Jan. 1996.

1 Hepatitis B (HB) may be given instead at 1-2 months, 4 months, 6-18 months. (A 3-dose series should be given by 12 years of age.)
2 Tetanus and diphtheria without Pertussis.
3 *H. influenzae type b* protects against several diseases, most notably meningitis. Shown is one schedule for Hib using one type of the vaccine. An alternate time schedule of 2, 4 and 12-15 months can be followed using a different form of the vaccine. Persons over 5 years of age are not given this vaccination unless sickle cell anemia or problems with the spleen are present.
4 The second dose of MMR vaccine should be given EITHER at 4-6 years OR at 11-12 years of age, depending on state school requirements.
5 Children who have not been vaccinated and who lack a reliable history of chicken pox should be vaccinated by 13 years of age. Children under 13 should get a single dose of VZV. Persons 13 and older should get two doses of VZV, 4-8 weeks apart.
6 Influenza vaccine may be recommended sooner than age 65 if you have a chronic medical condition such as diabetes mellitus, heart and/or respiratory diseases. Check with your doctor.
7 Pneumococcal vaccine may be recommended sooner than 65 if you have conditions that increase the risk of pneumonia such as chronic heart or lung disease, sickle cell disease, diabetes, Hodgkin's disease, or other conditions associated with a suppressed immune system.

Adult Immunizations

T(d)[2]	Tuberculin Tests	Influenza Vaccine (A&B)[6]	Pneumo-coccal Vaccine[7]
Every 10 years after 11-16 years of age	Upon Exposure	Annually After 65 Years	Once at 65 Years

Home Medical Tests

Medical self-testing kits are easy to use, relatively inexpensive, and readily available. They can be used without a visit to the doctor. It's no wonder that Americans are buying them more and more, spending over $500 million annually. Home tests can offer you a sense of self-reliance that can assist, though not take the place of, the service of your doctor.

While some 150 different medical self-testing kits exist, they generally can be grouped into two categories.

- Those that diagnose when conditions are or are not present. These include the popular self-testing kits for pregnancy, cholesterol, and kits that test for blood in the stool.
- Those that monitor an ongoing condition. These include blood sugar testing for diabetes and blood pressure kits for high blood pressure.

The U.S. Public Health Service and the Food and Drug Administration (FDA) offer some suggestions for safe and proper use of self-testing kits. (Each of these does not necessarily apply to all tests).

- For test kits that contain chemicals, note the expiration date. Beyond that date, chemicals may lose potency and affect results. Don't buy or use a test kit after the expiration date.
- Check whether the product needs protection from heat or cold. If so, don't leave it in the car trunk or by a sunny window on the trip home. At home, follow storage directions.
- Study the package insert. First, read it through to get a general idea of how to perform the test. Then, go back and review the instructions and diagrams until you fully understand each step.
- Be sure you understand what the test is intended to do and what its limitations may be. Remember, the tests are not 100 percent accurate.

- If the test results rely on color comparison and you're color blind, be sure someone is not color blind helps you interpret the results.
- Note special precautions, such as avoiding physical activity or certain foods and medications before testing.
- Follow instructions exactly, including the specimen collection process, if that is a part of the test. Sequence is important.
- Don't skip a step.
- When collecting a urine specimen (unless you use a container from a kit) wash the container thoroughly and rinse out all soap traces, preferably with distilled water.
- When a step is timed, be precise. Use a stopwatch, or at least a watch with a second hand.
- Note what you should do if the results are positive, negative, or unclear.
- If something isn't clear, don't guess. Consult a pharmacist or other health professional, or check the package for a toll-free "800" number to call for more information.
- Keep accurate records of results.
- As with medications, keep test kits that contain chemicals out of the reach of children. Throw away used test materials as directed.

Any malfunction of a self-test should be reported to the manufacturer or to the FDA through the agency's reporting system at the U.S. Pharmacopeia. To report a problem to the pharmacopeia, write to USP, Practitioner's Reporting Network, 12601 Twinbrook Parkway, Rockville, MD 20852. The report may also be called in toll-free at 1-800-638-6725.

chapter 3
MEDICATIONS

Before Taking Medications

Medications are powerful and can be harmful if not used properly. The tips below will help to reduce medicine related problems:

- Ask your doctor to not only tell you what a medicine is for, but ask him/her to write it down, too. If not, you might forget what the doctor says, especially if you're taking more than one medicine at a time. Your doctor should also tell you when to take it, for how long and if it should be taken in a special way, i.e., with food or plenty of water.

- Use the same pharmacy to buy prescriptions as well as over-the-counter medications. This way, a complete record of your medicines can be kept in one place. This is especially important if more than one doctor has been writing your prescriptions. Your pharmacist can also spot possible harmful combinations of medicines.

- Tell your doctor and have him/her record all medicines you take. This includes over-the-counter items like vitamins, aspirins, laxatives, etc., as well as any medicine another doctor has prescribed.

- Ask your pharmacists to clearly mark each vial with all necessary instructions.

- Always keep medicines in their original containers.

- Let your doctor know about your past reactions to certain medicines. Tolerance levels may change with age. For instance, as some people age, they may show greater sensitivity to some medications such as pain killers or tranquilizers.

- Ask about the possible side effects of a medication. If you do experience some, don't stop taking it, but call your physician immediately. Often, just a change in dosage is all that is needed.

- Never take someone else's medication.

- Throw away all medications that have expired.

- Try to reduce the need for medications, such as sleeping pills or laxatives. For example, a hot bath and a glass of milk might help you sleep at night. Changing your diet to increase your fiber intake might replace the need for a laxative. Even cutting down on salt and losing weight might lower blood pressure, avoiding the need for medication. Check with your doctor for non-medical alternatives.

- Don't stop taking medications your doctor has prescribed even if you feel better. Check with your physician first.

Understanding a Prescription

If you can't understand your doctor's prescription, much less read his/her handwriting, the following information will be helpful. Listed below are frequently used abbreviations that are meant to give directions to both the pharmacist filling the prescription and to the patient taking the medication.

ad lib. - Freely, as needed

a.c. - Before meals

b.i.d. - Twice a day

caps - Capsule

gtt. - Drops

h.s. - At bedtime

p.o. - By mouth

p.c. - After meals

p.r.n. - As needed

q.4.h. - Every 4 hours

q.i.d. - Four times a day

q.d. - Daily

q.o.d. - Every other day

t.i.d. - Three times a day

Ut dict., UD - As directed

Questions to Ask about Medications

Make sure you get clear answers to these questions before you take any medications.

- What is the name of the medicine?
- What will it do?
- When should it be taken?
- How long should it be taken?
- Are there side effects?
- Should I take it with meals?
- Is there a generic equivalent?
- Will it interfere with other medicines I am taking?
- Should I stop taking it if I feel better?
- Is there anything I should avoid while taking it? (Ex: Alcohol, sunlight, etc.)

Medication Match-Up

Categories of medicines and what they do are listed below.

Amphetamines - Stimulants that affect the central nervous system.

Analgesics - Pain relievers, such as aspirin.

Antacids - Relieve heartburn and indigestion by neutralizing stomach acid.

Antibiotics - Treat infections (usually bacterial ones).

Antiemetics - Treat nausea and vomiting.

Antihistamines - Used for colds or allergic reactions.

Barbituates - Sleep inducers.

Decongestants - Reduce swollen mucous membranes in the nose and sinuses.

Diuretics - Lower blood pressure by increasing the flow of urine.

Laxatives - Treat constipation.

Muscle Relaxants - Relieve muscle spasms.

Narcotics - Pain-killers and sleep-inducers that can be addictive.

Sedatives - Calming agents, tranquilizers or sleep inducers.

Other Medicine-Related Terms

Antiseptics - Destroy harmful germs.

Buffered - Antacids have been added to protect stomach lining.

Elixir - A liquid form of a medicine, that is usually pleasant tasting.

Generic - The name of a medicine that is available to be used by each drug manufacturer, often used to mean a less expensive equivalent of a brand name medicine.

7 Golden Rules of Prescriptions

Popping that pill into your mouth or spooning down that elixir may be hazardous to your health if you don't observe basic rules.

- ☐ Report adverse reactions, especially unexpected side effects, to your physician. Not everyone responds to medication in the same manner.

- ☐ Because two or more medications taken within a 24-hour period may interact negatively, tell your doctor about all medications you are taking. One medicine may slow down or speed up the effect of another. If you don't know which medications you take, bring them (in their original containers) with you to the doctor's office. Show them to your doctor.

- ☐ Ask your pharmacist about food and medication interactions. Some foods may affect the rate at which a medication works, or they can prevent it from working at all. Some combinations can have even more dangerous consequences. For example, when certain prescription medicines used to treat depression (MAO inhibitors) are consumed with cheese and other foods containing tyramine, dangerously elevated blood pressure levels may result.

- ☐ If you are having laboratory tests performed, be sure to inform the physician of all medications, nutritional supplements, etc., that you have been taking. Some of these substances can have an influence on certain test results. If you have administered a medical self-test, ask your pharmacist if anything you are taking will influence the test results.

- ☐ Don't drink alcohol while on a medication if you don't know its effect. Regular alcohol use can speed up the metabolism of certain medicines, reducing their intended effectiveness. When alcohol is present in the system, some medicines such as sedatives can become deadly.

- ☐ Always ask your physician if a generic equivalent would be okay to use. Generics are usually less expensive than the brand name item, and may be equally effective. There are certain situations in which a specific brand of medication may be required in order to ensure a consistent dosage. This is particularly important with medications for the heart, lung, and for hormonal disorders.

- ☐ Tell your doctor if:
  - You've ever experienced an allergic reaction, and to what.
  - You are pregnant or breast-feeding.
  - Another doctor is also treating you.
  - You have diabetes or kidney or liver disease.
  - You're regularly taking vitamins, birth control pills, insulin, or other medications.
  - You use alcohol, tobacco, or "street drugs."

Over-the-Counter Medications

Over-the-counter (OTC) medicines are widely advertised in magazines and on TV and are taken by millions of people. Generally less potent than prescription medicines, they can be taken without the authorization of a doctor. Ask these questions before buying an over-the-counter medicine:

☐ Am I trying to cover up symptoms that need to be evaluated by a doctor?

☐ Will continued use cause new problems (dependency on laxatives or sleeping pills, for example)?

☐ Are there unwanted side effects from these medicines (for example, increased blood pressure, dizziness, headaches, rashes)?

☐ Do I already have a similar product at home?

Often, reading the package labels or looking up the name of the medicine in the *Physician's Desk Reference for Nonprescription Drugs*, or asking the pharmacist can help you answer these questions. Keep in mind that when taken in large quantities, an OTC medicine might equal the dose of a medicine that is available only by prescription. If you are unsure whether or not a particular OTC medication will help or harm you, call and check with your doctor before you purchase it.

Overhauling Your Medicine Cabinet

Who knows what mysterious bottles lurk on the shelves of your bathroom medicine cabinet! If it has been more than a year since you last inventoried your cabinet, it's certainly time to do so. Here's how:

☐ Take out the entire contents of the medicine cabinet and get some clear idea of what you really need to keep.

☐ Check expiration dates. Throw out all outdated medicine. If you're uncertain about a particular item, call your pharmacist and ask what the shelf life is.

☐ Are all medications in original containers and labeled clearly? If not, into the trash they go. It's dangerous to store medicines in anything but their original containers. Some medicines come in tinted glass for example, because exposure to light may cause them to deteriorate.

☐ Discard old tubes of cream that have become hardened or cracked. Throw out any liquid medicines that now appear cloudy or filmy.

☐ If there are children in the house, every medication is a potential poison. Discard all unnecessary medications by flushing them down the toilet, and keep all others locked in a high cabinet, well out of their reach.

☐ Keep a container of Syrup of Ipecac* handy in case of accidental poisoning.

* *[Note: Call the poison control center before giving Syrup of Ipecac.]*

chapter 4
HOSPITALS & SURGERY

Ambulatory Surgery

Can you have surgery without being admitted to a hospital? Yes, and it's recommended in many cases. Ambulatory surgery can be done on an out-patient basis at a hospital or at facilities that perform out-patient surgeries. Procedures that best qualify for ambulatory surgery:

- ☐ Do not require opening a primary body section like the chest or skull.
- ☐ Do not require blood transfusions.
- ☐ Require very little or no general anesthesia.
- ☐ Do not require specialized postoperative care.
- ☐ Do not require hours on the operating table.
- ☐ Pose little risk of complication or additional surgery.

The most common types of surgeries performed in an ambulatory care center include:
- ☐ Hernia repair.
- ☐ Some plastic surgeries.
- ☐ Tubal ligation.
- ☐ Dilation and curettage (D and C).
- ☐ Breast biopsy.
- ☐ Tonsillectomy.
- ☐ Cataract removal.
- ☐ Adenoidectomy.
- ☐ Orthopedic procedures (such as setting a broken bone).
- ☐ Cystoscopy.
- ☐ Varicose vein surgery.
- ☐ Glaucoma procedures.

There are several important advantages of ambulatory or outpatient surgery.
- ☐ Hospitalization poses the risk of exposure to infection and may also keep patients bedridden longer than is necessary.
- ☐ Ambulatory surgery gets you in and out quickly.

- ☐ The patient has a good deal of choice as to when the surgery will occur. The surgeries are scheduled by appointment for patient convenience.
- ☐ Most people prefer healing at home in their own beds to staying in a hospital. Familiar surroundings and the comforts of home can be a more conducive environment in which to heal than the hectic schedules in many hospitals.
- ☐ Medical bills are much lower if you don't have to stay in a hospital overnight.

Things to consider:
- ☐ Many procedures require special preparation before the procedure. Follow your doctor's orders exactly.
- ☐ You may need someone to drive you home and stay with you as you recover.
- ☐ Do not bring valuables with you when you are admitted to the hospital.

Hospital Admissions

The golden rule here is to arrange for as much as you can before being admitted. Ask the following questions:
- ☐ Is it possible to have the needed forms mailed to your home prior to being admitted so that you may have the opportunity for careful review? Can you be "pre-admitted" over the telephone?
- ☐ Is your insurance coverage well understood both by the billing department and yourself?
- ☐ Can you reserve a private or semi-private room with your coverage?
- ☐ What identification will you need to have?
- ☐ Do you require special food preparations?

Medical Prefixes and Suffixes

Sometimes medical words require a "translation" into layman's terms. The following word beginnings and endings may help clarify the meanings of some medical terms.

Prefix	Definition	Example
angio-	blood vessels	angioplasty
arthro-	joint	arthroscopic
cardio-	heart	cardiovascular
cranio-	skull	cranioplasty
derma-	skin	dermatitis
gastro-	stomach	gastrointestinal
hem-	blood	hemophilia
hepato-	liver	hepatitis
myo-	muscle	myocardial
nephro-	kidney	nephritis
osteo-	bone	osteoporosis
radio-	ray	radiology
sacro-	sacrum	sacroiliac
uro-	urinary organs	uropenia
vaso-	vessel	vasoconstrictor

Suffix	Definition	Example
-algia or dynia	pain	neuralgia
-blast	early stage of a growth	cytotrophoblast
-ectomy	surgical removal	appendectomy
-itis	inflammation	bronchitis
-lysis	freeing of	dialysis
-oma	tumor	melanoma
-oscopy	viewing an organ	laparoscopy
-osis	process or condition	endometriosis
-otomy	cutting into	vasectomy
-pathy	abnormality	myopathy
-plasty	to rebuild or restore	rhinoplasty
-pnea	breathing	apnea
-rrhea	flow	diarrhea
-scler(osis)	hardening	arteriosclerosis
-uria	pertaining to urine	glycosuria

Saving Money in the Hospital

Avoid unnecessary stays in the hospital! The daily hospital rate in some sections of the country is now as high as $1,000.00. And that doesn't include the costs for treatments, medicines or doctor's fees. The hospital should never be viewed as a place to get a good rest. Consider these tips:

- ▢ Choose outpatient services whenever you can. Many routine lab tests and diagnostic tests and surgeries can be done for less money as an outpatient. You avoid the cost of an overnight stay in a hospital.

- ▢ As an inpatient, stay only the prescribed time that is necessary. Ask your doctor about home health care which can provide a whole range of services at less cost than in a hospital.

- ▢ Beware of duplication of tests. Be sure to ask the doctor about what blood tests, X-rays and medical procedures you can expect.

- ▢ Be sure you know when check out time is and make plans to observe it; otherwise, you're likely to be charged for an extra day's stay.

- ▢ If your health problem isn't an emergency, avoid being admitted to a hospital on a weekend. The hospital staff is reduced then, and testing will usually not begin until Monday.

- ▢ Same day or ambulatory surgery is a big money saver when compared to inpatient surgery. It can be used for minor procedures such as biopsies, cataract removal, etc.

- ▢ Keep a list of all services you receive in the hospital. Ask for an itemized bill so you can make sure you are billed correctly.

Types of Surgery

It's funny. People think of surgery as "major" when it happens to them and "minor" when it's being done to someone else! In reality, surgery is thought to be major when it involves any vital organs and/or requires a long time period to perform. The following chart helps to classify various surgeries.

Curative - A procedure that rids the body of a problem or corrects a condition.

Diagnostic - A procedure that helps in making a diagnosis about a suspected problem.

Elective - A procedure that may or may not be done, depending upon the patient's wishes.

Emergency - An immediate operation to save a life or maintain the use of a body part.

Exploratory - A surgery that explores a body organ or body area for a suspected disorder.

Palliative - A surgery that eases bodily pain, but doesn't cure the problem.

Planned - A surgery set up well in advance of the actual operation date.

Urgent - An operation that must be done within a matter of hours.

Patient Rights

What rights and privileges can you expect from a hospital when you become a patient? According to the American Hospital Association (AHA), there are specific standards of care that all patients are entitled to. The AHA has developed a voluntary code, The Patient's Bill of Rights, which presents guidelines for both staff and patients.

☐ You have the right to considerate and respectful care.

☐ You have the right to obtain from your physician complete, current information concerning your diagnosis, treatment, and prognosis in terms you can reasonably be expected to understand.

☐ You have the right to receive from your physician information necessary to give informed consent prior to the start of any procedure and/or treatment.

☐ You have the right to refuse treatment to the extent permitted by law, and to be informed of the medical consequences of your action.

☐ You have the right to privacy concerning your own medical care program, including all communications and records pertaining to your care.

☐ You have the right to expect that within its capacity a hospital must make a reasonable response to your request for services.

☐ You have the right to obtain information about any relationship of your hospital to other health care and educational institutions insofar as your care is concerned.

☐ You have the right to be advised if the hospital proposes to engage in or perform human experimentation affecting your care or treatment.

☐ You have the right to expect reasonable continuity of care.

☐ You have the right to examine and receive an explanation of your bill regardless of the source of payment.

☐ You have the right to know what hospital rules and regulations apply to your conduct as a patient.

Informed Consent

Every patient should be aware of the policy of informed consent, an ethical standard in medicine that implies that you have been given an explanation and fully understand your treatment. You should be able to explain in your own words what your treatment is about. You should know what the likelihood is that the medical procedure will accomplish what it's supposed to. The benefits and the accompanying risks should always be identified clearly. You should also be notified if your treatment is experimental in nature.

The physician should review any alternatives that are available in lieu of surgery or other procedures. There is no guaranteed outcomes in medicine, but informed consent enables YOU to make a rational and educated decision about your treatment. It is also a tool that promotes greater understanding between you and your doctor and encourages joint decision making.

Three principles of informed consent that involve your responsibility as a patient are:

- You cannot demand services that go beyond what are considered "acceptable" practices of medicine or that violate professional ethics.
- You must recognize that you may be faced with some uncertainties or unpleasantness.
- You should, if competent, be responsible for your choices. Don't have others make decisions for you.

Advance Directives

A federal law called the Patient Self Determination Act requires hospitals and nursing homes to give you information about your rights to refuse treatment under state law. Advance directives are a legal way for you to declare your wishes regarding the withholding or removal of life sustaining care if you should suffer from a terminal illness, or if you should be in an incurable or irreversible mental or physical condition with no reasonable expectations of recovery.

There are two types of advance directives:

- Living Will - A document that spells out what medical treatment you would want or not want if you are unable to state it yourself. Most states have their own Living Will form or you can make up your own. You should discuss your living will with your family and physician.
- Durable Power of Attorney (Health-Care Proxy)- A document that names a person who would make treatment decisions for you if you are not able to make them yourself. Generally, it is a person who knows you and your values well and is in a good position to represent your wishes to your physician.

chapter 5
HEALTH INSURANCE

Insurance Terms

Does it seem to you that health insurance policies are written in something other than simple English. Here are some terms that will help you understand a policy.

Assigned Benefits - The doctor accepts payment directly from the insurance company.

Co-insurance - Means you pay a certain percentage (usually 20%) of the costs of a service. There may or may not be a set limit, after which the insurance coverage is 100%.

Co-payment - Cost sharing requirement in many health insurance policies, in which the insured pays a percentage of or pre-set fee for the cost of covered services.

Covered Expenses - Medical expenses that are paid for under the terms of a policy.

Deductible - The amount of money you must pay for medical expenses before the company pays anything.

Exclusion - A service that health insurance company will not cover or pay for.

Pre-authorization - A requirement that calls for approval ahead of time from the insurance company for certain services specified in the policy.

Pre-existing Condition - A health problem you had when the insurance took effect.

Stop-loss - A provision that limits the amount you make in co-payments to a maximum figure.

Usual and Customary - Stands for the usual fees charged for medical services.

Waiting Period - The period during which an insurance policy will not cover a problem.

Considering Your Needs

The right health insurance for you depends on your needs and the needs of your family. Policies vary, therefore, as do costs and what is covered. Be a wise shopper. Consider your needs before choosing health insurance. Ask these questions:

- Is my whole family covered?
- Are most services covered?
- Are routine checkups covered?
- Are well-care visits covered?
- Are immunizations covered?
- Is maternity care covered?
- Are there deductibles? What are they?
- Are there limits if my problem is chronic?
- How many days are covered in the hospital?
- Are psychological services covered?
- Can I choose my doctor? Can I be seen by the same doctor at each visit?
- Are specialist visits covered?

It's best to talk to someone who knows a lot about health insurance for advice. Just because a friend, relative, or fellow employee chooses a certain health insurance policy, doesn't mean it's right for you. Also, ask your employee benefits person or Employee Assistance Program (EAP) representative for information on health insurance your company offers.

chapter 6
MEDICAL DECISIONS

At some point in your life (maybe it's right now), you or a loved one may be faced with making a medical decision that could affect your quality of life. You can deal with this issue with greater ease when you have all the information you need. One way to get this information is to ask your doctor all the right questions. This section will teach you what to ask.

Key Questions Checklist

(Photocopy as needed)

The following is a summary of the key questions and recommendations that will assist you in making medical decisions. Use them as a guide when visiting your doctor or health care professional. Check off the items you wish to discuss with your doctor or health care professional as the need arises.

1. **Description - What is my current complaint?**
   - ❑ What do I think the problem is?
   - ❑ When did it start?
   - ❑ What makes it better?
   - ❑ What makes it worse?
   - ❑ What are my signs and symptoms?
   - ❑ What daily habits are affected (i.e., eating, sleeping, activity, etc.). Is it consistent or only at certain times?

2. **Diagnosis - What is my diagnosis?**
   - ❑ Can you explain the diagnosis to me in detail?
   - ❑ Is my condition chronic or acute?
   - ❑ If it is chronic, how will it affect my life?
   - ❑ Is my condition one that will be with me constantly or will it come and go?
   - ❑ If it will come and go, how often should I expect it?
   - ❑ Is there anything I can do to help prevent it?
   - ❑ Is my condition contagious? If yes, what should I do?
   - ❑ Is my condition genetic? If yes, what can I do?
   - ❑ How certain are you about this diagnosis?
   - ❑ Do you have any literature about my condition?
   - ❑ Is there a support group available?

3. **Treatment - What is the recommended treatment plan?**
   - ❑ Write down a description of the recommended treatment plan.
   - ❑ What results do you expect?
   - ❑ When can I expect to see results?

If you are discussing surgery:
   - ❑ Give me a step-by-step account of the procedure, including anesthesia and recovery. Also, consider getting a second opinion.

If you are discussing a test:
   - ❑ What is the test called and how will it help identify what is wrong?
   - ❑ Will it give us specific or general information?
   - ❑ If the answer is general, where do we go from here?
   - ❑ Will more tests be necessary?
   - ❑ How accurate and reliable is the test?
   - ❑ Is the test invasive or non-invasive?
   - ❑ What will I have to do to prepare for the test?
   - ❑ Where do I go for the test?
   - ❑ How and when will I get the test's results?

(Also see "Questions to Ask about Medications" on page 21).

4. **Benefits - What are the benefits of the treatment?**
   - ❑ What will be the specific benefits if I go ahead with the treatment?
   - ❑ To what extent will the treatment improve my condition?
   - ❑ Is there documented evidence the recommended treatment will have a positive outcome?

5. **Risks - What are the potential risks of the treatment?**
   - ❑ List the possible risks and complications.
   - ❑ Do the benefits outweigh the risks or vice-versa?
   - ❑ Make a list of the risks and benefits rating each between one and five to aid in your decision-making process. (One being not as important, and five being very important).

6. **Success - What is the success rate for the treatment?**
   - ❑ What is the national success rate?
   - ❑ What is the success rate at the hospital/medical facility where my treatment is planned?
   - ❑ What is the surgeon's success rate and experience with the surgery?
   - ❑ How many procedures are the above success rates based on?
   - ❑ Are there any personal factors that will affect my odds either way?
   - ❑ How long will the results of my surgery/treatment last?

7. **Timing - When should I begin the treatment?**
   - ❑ When is the best time to get started with the treatment plan?
   - ❑ Do I have to undergo treatment right away? If not, how long can I safely wait?
   - ❑ Determine the best time for you to begin the treatment plan.

8. **Alternatives - What are my options?**
   - ❑ What will happen if I decide to do nothing?
   - ❑ What are my other options? Include non-surgical and outpatient alternatives if you are discussing surgery.
   - ❑ If you are not satisfied with your options, discuss this with your doctor. If you are still not satisfied, you may consider consulting another physician.
   - ❑ Investigate every option which you are considering as thoroughly as the original treatment plan.

9. **Cost - How much will the treatment cost?**
   - ❑ What is the cost of the recommended treatment plan?
   - ❑ Check with your insurance company to see what portion will be covered and whether you need to do anything to receive maximum coverage, i.e., seeking a second opinion, getting pre-authorization, etc.
   - ❑ What related costs do I need to consider, i.e., time off work, child care, transportation, etc.?

10. **Decision - What do I decide to do?**
    - ❑ You are now in a better position to make an intelligent, informed decision.
    - ❑ Remember, you are ultimately responsible for your body and have the right to choose or refuse treatment.
    - ❑ If you feel rushed or otherwise uncomfortable when discussing this information with your doctor, tell him or her how you feel.

Medical Decision Comparison Chart

(Photocopy as needed)

Use this chart to help you compare different medical options that are available to you.

Diagnosis _____

	Option One		Option Two		Option Three	
Treatment						
Benefits						
Risks						
Success						
Timing						
Alternatives						
Cost						
Decision	Yes ❑	No ❑	Yes ❑	No ❑	Yes ❑	No ❑

Wallet Size Checklist

1. **Diagnosis**
   - ❑ What is my diagnosis?
   - ❑ Is my condition chronic or acute?
   - ❑ Is my condition one that will be with me constantly?
   - ❑ Is there anything I can do to help prevent it?
   - ❑ Is my condition contagious or genetic?
   - ❑ How certain are you about this diagnosis?
2. **Treatment**
   - ❑ What is the recommended treatment?

   If you are discussing medications:
   - ❑ What will the medicine do for my particular problem?
   - ❑ When, how often and for how long should I take the medicine?
   - ❑ How long before the medicine starts working?
   - ❑ Will there be side effects?
   - ❑ Will there be interactions with other medications I am taking?

If you are discussing a test:
   - ❑ What is the test called and how will it help identify the problem?
   - ❑ Will it give us specific or general information?
   - ❑ Will more tests be necessary?
   - ❑ How accurate and reliable is the test?
   - ❑ How should I prepare for the test?
   - ❑ Where do I go for the test?
   - ❑ How and when will I get the test's results?

If you are discussing surgery:
   - ❑ Will you give me a step-by-step account of the procedure, including anesthesia and recovery?
3. **Benefits vs. Risks**
   - ❑ What are the benefits if I go ahead with the treatment?
   - ❑ What are the possible risks and complications?
   - ❑ Do the benefits outweigh the risks or vice-versa?
4. **Success**
   - ❑ What is the success rate for the treatment?
   - ❑ Are there any personal factors that will affect my odds either way?

   - ❑ How long will the results of my treatment last?
5. **Timing**
   - ❑ When is the best time to begin the treatment?
   - ❑ When can I expect to see results?
6. **Alternatives**
   - ❑ What will happen if I decide to do nothing?
   - ❑ What are my other options?
7. **Cost**
   - ❑ What is the cost of the recommended treatment?
   - ❑ What related costs should I consider, i.e., time off work, child care, travel, etc.?
8. **Decision**
   - ❑ You can now make an informed decision.
   - ❑ Remember, you have the right to choose or refuse treatment.
   - ❑ If you feel rushed or uncomfortable when talking with your doctor, tell him or her how you feel.

chapter 7
YOU AND YOUR DENTIST

An overall picture of a healthy person is incomplete if it doesn't include the vital role of proper dental care and good oral hygiene. A family dentist who is knowledgeable and prevention oriented is a valued part of everyone's health care team.

The Dental Checkup

The following components insure a proper examination of your mouth by a dentist.

- Visual check of the soft tissues (tongue, cheek, throat and gums) for redness and puffiness, or white discoloration.
- Check the bite and jaw joints.
- Measure any pockets which may have developed between the teeth and the gums. (This is a check for periodontal problems).
- Full set of X-rays (if they haven't been taken recently).
- Asking the patient about any areas of concern.

When to Visit Your Dentist

- Every six months for a cleaning and checkup.
- If your gums bleed easily or are swollen, reddened or soft.
- If you notice a change in your bite.
- If you have an injury to a tooth or it is dislodged due to an accident. (It can often be replanted if seen by a dentist immediately).
- If you have any discomfort from a tooth.
- If you have a tendency to grind your teeth, experience pain near the jaw joint, or have chronic headaches.

Dental Specialties

The American Dental Association recognizes a number of different dental specialties:

Endodontics - disease prevention and treatment of root pulp (the living tissue that conveys sensation to the tooth).

Oral Surgeon (Maxillofacial Surgeon) - surgical treatment of jaw and mouth injuries, diseases or tooth extraction.

Orthodontics - correcting mouth deformities or tooth irregularities, often through braces or functional appliances.

Pedodontics - care of children's teeth.

Periodontics - preventive care and treatment of structures that surround and support the teeth (Ex: Gums).

Prosthodontics - rehabilitation of oral problems with such devices as bridges, crowns, or dentures.

Public Health Dentistry - control of dental disease through community dental programs.

All of these specialties require at least two additional years of advanced training after dental school.

chapter 8
MENTAL HEALTH

People who are mentally healthy feel good about themselves and comfortable with others. They are also able to deal with the demands, challenges, and changes in everyday life.

Everyone, regardless of age, race, sex, or economic status, is subject to emotional upsets. You can feel down, angry, or anxious in response to a variety of things. Feelings like these can come and go quite often. When these feelings are disturbing, interfere with daily life, and/or linger for weeks or months, they may signal a problem that requires professional assistance. According to the National Institute for Mental Health (NIMH), at any given time, approximately 40 million Americans (about 1 in 6) experience a mental disorder that interferes with employment and/or daily life.

Mental Health Facts

- About 25% of the people who seek medical help for physical problems actually have troubled emotions.
- The most common reasons people seek mental health treatment are for depression and anxiety.
- Between 8 and 14 million Americans suffer from depression each year.
- Approximately 80 to 90% of all depressed people respond to treatment.
- Approximately 10% of Americans have phobias.
- 12.5 million Americans are drug abusers or are chemically dependent.
- 13 million are dependent on alcohol. (This includes 3 million children).
- Nearly 25% of the elderly who are thought to be senile actually suffer some form of mental illness that can be treated effectively.
- Therapy does not have to take a long time. Almost one-half of the people who enter therapy will complete it in seven sessions or less.

It's Smart to Ask for Help

Many people are reluctant to seek mental health services because of the "stigma" of having an "emotional" problem. Society has a tendency to view mental health issues differently from medical ones. When someone breaks a leg, has chest pains, or needs to get a prescription, they'll see a doctor. However, when they experience depression, excessive fears, or a problem with alcohol, they may be embarrassed to seek help. Many people view these conditions as "weaknesses" that they should be able to handle themselves. Unfortunately, this view keeps them from getting professional help that can help them deal with and/or treat these conditions.

To recognize a problem and receive psychological help is not a sign of weakness at all. Rather, to do so is a sign of strength. Also, taking part in your company's Employee Assistance Program (EAP) or seeing a therapist is completely confidential. No information will be released to anyone without your permission.

Reasons to Seek Help

The following symptoms usually signal the need for professional help. Only a trained professional can diagnose and determine the treatment needed.

- ☐ Thinking or talking about suicide.
- ☐ Seeing or hearing things that aren't actually present.
- ☐ Suspiciousness or paranoia.
- ☐ Strange or grandiose ideas.
- ☐ Crippling or excessive anxieties (phobias or fears).
- ☐ Wide mood swings (extreme highs and lows).
- ☐ Prolonged depression and apathy (a sense of hopelessness, loss of pleasure in life, confusion or constant frustration).
- ☐ Marked personality change.
- ☐ Compulsive behaviors (i.e., over spending, overeating, excessive exercising).
- ☐ Marked changes in eating or sleeping patterns.
- ☐ Excessive anger or hostility; destructive, abusive or violent behavior.
- ☐ Problems with the law.
- ☐ Difficulty with authority.
- ☐ Abuse of alcohol and/or other drugs.
- ☐ Difficulty interacting with other people (spouse, parents, children, co-workers, and friends).
- ☐ Denial of obvious problems; strong resistance to receiving help.
- ☐ Social withdrawal and isolation.
- ☐ Inability to cope with the loss of a loved one.
- ☐ Extreme jealousy.
- ☐ Preoccupation with physical illness.
- ☐ Overall decline in job performance.
- ☐ Problems on the job.
- ☐ A feeling that you've lost control of your life.
- ☐ Inability to cope with problems or daily activities such as school, job or personal needs.
- ☐ Sexual problems.

Common Mental Health Conditions

Anxiety Disorder - Characterized by unrealistic or excessive worry about any real or imagined life circumstances (i.e., finances, social performance). Persons experiencing anxiety may have rapid pulse and/or breathing rate, racing or pounding heart, dry mouth, sweating, trembling, shaking, shortness of breath, faintness, tension, or stomach problems.

Bipolar Disorder (Manic-Depression) - A mood disorder characterized by mood swings from elation and/or euphoria to severe depression. Extreme irritability is common during the euphoric phase of the disease. A phase can last anywhere from several days to several months before another mood swing. It usually occurs before the age of 35 and affects one percent of the population at some time in their lives.

Critical Incident Stress Syndrome - Psychological symptoms and/or physical conditions caused by a specific traumatic event. Examples include workplace traumas such as threatened or actual acts of violence and injury or death. It is similar to Post Traumatic Stress Syndrome where people who have experienced a critical event often suffer from acute anxiety, depression, and feeling out of control. They may also have nightmares and/or flashbacks of the event.

Dependent Personality - Characterized by dependent and submissive behavior. This person has difficulty making decisions without a tremendous amount of advice from others. Persons with dependent personalities will even allow others to make important decisions for them and are overly concerned with other people liking them.

Depression - A condition marked by sadness, hopelessness, helplessness, pessimism, and a loss of interest in life. Symptoms of depression include long-lasting crying spells, fatigue, loss of interest or pleasure in ordinary activities including sex, changes in eating and sleeping patterns, lack of concentration, and thoughts of suicide or death.

Hypochondria - A condition characterized by a preoccupation with one's health. People with hypochondria falsely believe they have some disease, even though physical examinations show otherwise.

Histrionic Personality - A condition characterized by a consistent pattern of being excessively emotional to get attention. Histrionics put excessive focus on intimate relationships and material things.

Jealousy - Normal jealousy is usually a harmless condition in which people feel someone or something they like or love might be taken away by another person. Excessive jealousy, however, is an intense, mentally painful condition which causes the sufferer to become suspicious and always be on the look-out for signs that they are losing the person or object they desire. These people become obsessed with their fears and often cannot concentrate on anything else

Narcissistic Personality - This disorder is characterized by an excessive sense of self-importance. Narcissists exaggerate their accomplishments and abilities and expect to be viewed as special even if their achievements do not warrant it.

Obsessive-Compulsive Disorder - An anxiety disorder where the sufferer has persistent, involuntary thoughts or images (obsessions) and engages in ritualistic acts such as washing their hands according to certain self-imposed rules (compulsions).

Panic Attack - A brief period of acute anxiety that can occur without warning. Symptoms include shortness of breath, chest discomfort, heart palpitations, sweating, and choking.

Paranoid Personality - A pattern of thinking and behaving characterized by suspiciousness, mistrust of others, and over-sensitivity. These people make an effort to find evidence that confirms their prejudices or attitudes.

Passive-Aggressive Personality - Describes people who are both passive and aggressive at the same time. They express their hostility in indirect and non-violent ways such as procrastinating, forgetting, habitual tardiness, and lying. They resent anyone making demands of them and, through their aggravating behavior, make sure they do not comply with these demands.

Phobia - An anxiety disorder, where the individual feels terror, dread or panic when faced with a feared object, situation, or activity. Examples include simple phobias, such as being afraid of snakes, social phobias, such as the fear of speaking in front of other people and complex phobias, such as agoraphobia, which is the fear of being in places or situations from which escape might be difficult or embarrassing).

Post-Traumatic Stress Syndrome - A condition where a person re-experiences a traumatic past event like a wartime situation, hostage-taking, or rape. Symptoms include nightmares, flashbacks of the event, excessive alertness, and emotional numbness to people and activities.

Schizophrenia - A group of mental disorders in which there are severe disturbances in thinking, mood, and behavior. The sufferer experiences delusions, hallucinations, disordered thinking, and/or inappropriate emotions.

Substance Abuse - Misuse of drugs (both legal and illegal) and/or alcohol on a regular basis even though doing so interferes with daily life.

chapter 9
STAYING WELL

A new interest is taking hold today: The interest people have in making themselves healthy. The American public, in greater numbers than ever before, want to do those things that will promote health longevity, and increase the quality of life. Exercise gyms are booming, health foods are readily accessible, cigarette smoking is the exception and not the rule, and you can hardly go anywhere without seeing joggers trot by. We have come a long way from Mark Twain's philosophy that "The only way to keep your health is to eat what you don't want, drink what you don't like and do what you'd rather not."

It's encouraging to see people's desire to make their lifestyle the best it can be! The emphasis is also shifting from traditional medicine, which is designed to treat illness, to doing those things that prevent sickness from occurring in the first place. The public wants to become better health consumers as well. We recognize warning signs. We read labels. We know when a doctor is or is not needed. We are opening our eyes to the risk factors for conditions such as heart disease, diabetes, and cancer.

This chapter deals with eight topics that are important to good health as well as to preventing disease.

Cigarette Smoking: Packing it In

It is not easy to quit smoking cigarettes. This is because smoking involves both physical and psychological components. Nicotine is a physically addictive substance. After an initial rejection by the body, a tolerance level develops in the smoker, and withdrawal symptoms occur when nicotine is withheld. Cigarettes also produce a psychological dependence. The desire to smoke is "triggered" by certain situations, emotions, and a need to inhale and exhale on something.

Smoking Facts

- Cigarette smoking is our nation's #1 preventable cause of illness and premature death. Over 440,000 people in the U.S. die from the effects of smoking each year.
- After inhaling, 70-90% of the chemical compounds in a cigarette stay in the smoker's lungs.
- Cigarette smokers are 15 times more likely to get lung cancer, 16 times more likely to have emphysema, 10 times more likely to have bronchitis, and twice as likely to have a heart attack than nonsmokers.
- Nonsmokers who inhale second hand smoke from a burning cigarette have an increased risk of lung cancer and heart disease as well.
- Pregnant women who smoke are cutting off oxygen to their developing fetus as well as altering the blood pressure and heart rate of the baby. Low birth weights, spontaneous abortions and stillbirths are more prevalent in smokers.
- Medical research has found that each cigarette smoked takes 15 minutes off one's life.
- Children of smokers have twice the incidence of respiratory ailments as the children of nonsmokers.
- According to the American Cancer Society, eight out of ten smokers would like to quit.

The "Warm Pheasant" Plan to Quit Smoking

You've heard of quitting cigarettes cold turkey, all at once, in an unflinching moment of resolution. Well, that works for some, but not all, smokers. In fact, there are as many ways to quit smoking as there are brands of cigarettes for sale. If you're like Mark Twain who said, "Quitting smoking is easy. I've done it over a hundred times", you might want to try the "warm pheasant" method. Unlike the cold turkey approach, this three-phase plan allows you to continue to smoke, while you prepare to quit, psychologically and physically.

Phase I: Preparing to Quit

This phase takes approximately one week.

- ☐ Mark a "quit" date on your calendar one week in advance.
- ☐ Keep track of each cigarette you smoke by making a slash mark on a piece of paper tucked in the wrapper of your cigarette pack.
- ☐ Every time you have an urge to light up, wait 10 minutes.
- ☐ Collect your cigarette butts in a "butt bottle." (The mere sight of so many spent cigarettes will graphically demonstrate just how much you really smoke in a week).

Phase II: Quitting

This phase takes approximately one to two weeks.

- ☐ Throw away all your cigarettes and hide all smoking paraphernalia, like matches, lighters, ashtrays, and so forth.
- ☐ Whenever you have an urge to smoke, take a deep breath through your mouth and slowly exhale through pursed lips. Repeat five to ten times.
- ☐ Change your routine to eliminate familiar smoking cues. If you always light up when driving to work, take a different route. Or substitute a walk for your usual coffee-and cigarette break. Or sit in a chair you don't customarily use when relaxing or watching television at home.
- ☐ Take up activities you don't normally associate with smoking. Enroll in a cooking class, visit a non-smoking friend, or go swimming at your local Y, for example.

- ☐ Keep your hands busy by holding something, such as a pen, Nerf Ball, or a binder clip.
- ☐ In place of cigarettes, substitute other things that will provide oral gratification, like sugarless gum or mints, toothpicks, or coffee stirrers.
- ☐ Avoid drinking coffee and alcohol or eating foods high in sugar, like candy and pastries. They cause biochemical changes in the body that increase your desire for a cigarette.
- ☐ Create a "piggy bank" and put the money you used to spend on cigarettes in a jar. Watch it add up.
- ☐ Place a rubber band on your wrist and snap it every time you get an urge to smoke.

Phase III: Staying off Cigarettes

Allow three months for this final phase.

- ☐ Always remember that the craving to smoke will pass, whether you smoke or not.
- ☐ Renew your commitment to stay off cigarettes each day.
- ☐ Beware of saboteurs, usually other smokers, who may try to encourage you to light up. Assert your right to not smoke.
- ☐ Talk to a non-smoking buddy for support.
- ☐ Make a list of good things you've noticed since you quit, e.g., food tastes better, you cough less, your clothes don't smell bad, and so forth.
- ☐ Continue to practice the behavior modification techniques listed in the quitting phase.

SOURCE: The Smokeless Program, the American Institute for Preventive Medicine, Farmington Hills, Michigan, 1994.

Stress - Learning to Cope

Do you know what stress is?

- ▭ Stress is the body's non-specific response to any increased demand placed upon it.
- ▭ Stressors are those events, objects or thoughts that will cause the stress response to occur.

Keeping Track of Stress Signals

Many of us have symptoms of stress every day without realizing it. To recognize the signals your body is sending you, read this partial list of stress symptoms. Make a mental note or place a check next to those symptoms that you've experienced when under stress. Place two checks if you experience this symptom frequently. Write in any other symptoms you experience when feeling stressed. *[Note: Symptoms of stress could indicate a physical problem and should be checked out before assuming you are not coping well.]*

Symptoms of Stress

▭ Nervous tic	▭ Jittery feelings
▭ Clearing throat	▭ Rapid heartbeat
▭ Clenching hands	▭ Sweating
▭ Gritting teeth	▭ Sexual difficulties
▭ Feeling lonely	▭ Dry mouth and throat
▭ Queasy stomach	▭ Irritability
▭ Vomiting	▭ Emotional instability
▭ Diarrhea	▭ Inability to concentrate
▭ Headache	▭ Accident proneness
▭ Backache	▭ Stuttering
▭ Neck ache	▭ Insomnia
▭ Hives	▭ Forgetfulness
▭ Constipation	▭ Frequent urination
▭ Depression	▭ Nightmares
▭ Rash	▭ Negative thoughts
▭ Pacing	▭ Faintness or dizziness
▭ Foot tapping	▭ Lack of interest
▭ Overeating	▭ Low energy level
▭ Smoking	▭ Temper outbursts
▭ Drinking	▭ _____
▭ Feeling fearful	▭ _____
▭ Crying	▭ _____
▭ Fatigue	▭ _____

Conditions Related to Stress

Research has revealed a clear link between physical illness and stress. In some cases, stress plays an important part in the nature and severity of the illness. In fact, the American Academy of Family Physicians states that approximately two thirds of all visits to the family doctor are for stress related disorders. Read the list below. Make additions if you feel that stress contributes to a condition that is not listed.

Conditions Associated with or Made Worse by Stress

▭ Acne	▭ Low back pain
▭ Alcoholism	▭ Lowering of the
▭ Allergies	body's immune
▭ Arthritis	systems
▭ Asthma	▭ Nervous
▭ Backaches	breakdown
▭ Cancer	▭ Neurosis
▭ Colitis	▭ Premenstrual
▭ Common cold	syndrome (PMS)
▭ Coronary heart	▭ Stroke
disease	▭ Temporal Mandibular
▭ Eating disorders	Joint Syndrome (TMJ)
▭ Eczema	▭ _____
▭ Gout	▭ _____
▭ Headaches	▭ _____
▭ High blood pressure	▭ _____
▭ Insomnia	▭ _____

Life Events Questionnaire

Is there a connection between the number of major life events a person experiences in a year and the likelihood of illness? Drs. Thomas Holmes and Richard Rahe think so. They reached this conclusion after questioning 7,000 people about the number of life events they went through in one year. The people who scored highest on this questionnaire experienced the highest amount of physical illness in the year following the test. Since major life changes can produce stress-induced illness, take a look at how the past year's life events add up for you.

Instructions

Place a check mark in the column labeled 'Happened" for those events that occurred in the past 12 months. Then record your score with the event value for each. Total the score for each column, and then add those totals to get a grand total.

Event Rank	Event Value	Hap-pened	Your Score	Life Event	Event Rank	Event Value	Hap-pened	Your Score	Life Event
1	100	___	___	Death of a spouse	23	29	___	___	Son or daughter leaving home
2	73	___	___	Divorce	24	29	___	___	Trouble with in-laws
3	65	___	___	Marital separation	25	28	___	___	Outstanding personal
4	63	___	___	Jail term					achievement
5	63	___	___	Death of close family	26	26	___	___	Spouse begins or stops work
				member	27	26	___	___	Begin or end of school
6	53	___	___	Personal injury or illness	28	25	___	___	Change of living conditions
7	50	___	___	Marriage	29	24	___	___	Revision of personal habits
8	47	___	___	Fired from job	30	23	___	___	Trouble with boss
9	45	___	___	Marital reconciliation	31	20	___	___	Change in work hours or
10	45	___	___	Retirement					conditions
11	44	___	___	Change in health of	32	20	___	___	Change in residence
				family member	33	20	___	___	Change in schools
12	40	___	___	Pregnancy	34	19	___	___	Change in recreation
13	39	___	___	Sex difficulties	35	19	___	___	Change in church activities
14	39	___	___	Gain of new family	36	18	___	___	Change in social activities
				member	37	17	___	___	Mortgage or loan less than
15	39	___	___	Business readjustment					$50,000*
16	39	___	___	Change in financial state	38	16	___	___	Change in sleeping habits
17	37	___	___	Death of close friend	39	15	___	___	Change in number of family
18	36	___	___	Change line of work					get-togethers
19	35	___	___	Change number of arguments	40	15	___	___	Change in eating habits
				with spouse	41	13	___	___	Vacation
20	31	___	___	Mortgage over $50,000*	42	12	___	___	Christmas
21	30	___	___	Foreclosure of mortgage/ loan	43	11	___	___	Minor violations of the law
22	29	___	___	Change in duties at work				___	**TOTAL COLUMN 2**
			___	**TOTAL COLUMN 1**				+ ___	**TOTAL COLUMN 1**
								___	**GRAND TOTAL**

* The financial amount was increased by $40,000 from the original Life Events Questionnaire to reflect current economic conditions.
1976, Thomas Holmes, M.D., and Richard Rahe, Ph.D.

Scoring

- People who score between 100-199 have a very mild risk.
- People who score between 200-299 have a more moderate risk of developing physical illness in the next 12 months.
- People who score 300 or more have a strong risk of developing physical illness in the next 12 months.

[Note: These scores only represent a likelihood of getting sick and not a definite prediction.]

Tips for Stress Management

- Maintain a regular program of healthy eating, good health habits, and adequate sleep.
- Exercise regularly. This promotes physical fitness and emotional well being.
- Don't let your emotions get "bottled up" inside. Share your feelings with others.
- Learn to manage your time efficiently.
- Avoid unnecessary arguments or quarrels.
- Do a "stress rehearsal." Prepare for stressful events by imagining yourself feeling calm and handling the situation well.
- Minimize your exposure to things that cause distress.
- Practice a relaxation technique daily.
- Several times a day, do a "body check" for tensed muscles and let them relax.
- Do deep breathing exercises.
- Be a good Samaritan. Spend time helping others.
- Balance work and play.
- Plan some "me" time daily.
- Engage in activities you enjoy and look forward to.
- Discover the "elf" in yourself. Learn to have fun.
- He who laughs, lasts. Improve your laugh life.
- Participate in activities with people who share your interests.
- Reward yourself with little things that make you feel good.
- Challenge yourself to do something new.
- Surround yourself with cheery people. Avoid stress carriers.
- Shun the "superman" or "superwoman" syndrome. No one is perfect.
- Set realistic goals for yourself.
- Be flexible in dealing with people and events.
- Avoid "psychosclerosis" - a hardening of the attitudes.
- Accept the things you cannot change in yourself or others.
- Forgive yourself for mistakes.
- Take satisfaction in your accomplishments. Don't dwell on your shortcomings.
- Develop and maintain a positive attitude. View changes as positive challenges, opportunities or blessings.
- Seek professional help if needed.

Fitness - Get Fit, Stay Fit

Physical fitness has many benefits:

- ▭ Stress, boredom and depression are minimized as exercise seems to take the edge off daily tension.
- ▭ Skin tone is improved through fitness . . . giving that healthy glow!
- ▭ When our bodies demand more oxygen, such as for climbing stairs, it's no problem!
- ▭ Muscle tone is revitalized; strength, endurance and even posture can improve.
- ▭ Fitness allows your heart to function with less strain placed upon it.
- ▭ Our self-esteem tends to improve as we see good things in the mirror!
- ▭ Blood circulation gets better and better.
- ▭ We sleep better.
- ▭ Our appetite for food is more manageable and our digestive process works better.
- ▭ Greater flexibility and ease are seen in the joints. Fewer creaks!
- ▭ Physical exercise increases the number of calories that are burned. In fact, calories are burned at a 15% higher rate for up to 6 hours after activity.

Beginning an Exercise Program

There are some basic points to keep in mind when beginning an exercise program:

- ▭ Before beginning to exercise, it is advisable that you consult your physician, particularly if you have been inactive for an extended period of time, are overweight, are over 35 years old, and/or have a medical problem.
- ▭ Choose an activity plan that is right for you. Take into consideration where it will be done, what equipment is needed, whether it will be done with others, if it can be done in bad weather, what the cost is, and most importantly, whether you will enjoy it.

- ▭ Ease into your exercise program. Start off with activities of low intensity, frequency, and duration. Then build up your pace over the next several weeks. A good rule to follow is that if you can't talk while exercising, you're overdoing it.
- ▭ Do warm up exercises before the activity. Loosen up your muscles by stretching and/or walking for 5 minutes. When the activity is done, cool down with 5 more minutes of walking and/or stretching.
- ▭ Select an appropriate time and place to do your exercise. Get into a routine where the activity is done at the same time each day. Wait at least 2 hours after eating before doing a strenuous activity. If you exercise before a meal, wait about 25 minutes before you eat.
- ▭ For good results you should exercise at least three times a week for at least 20 minutes.
- ▭ Be in tune with your body while exercising. If muscles or joints start to hurt, ease up. It is usually not necessary to stop all activity for minor soreness. Be aware of the warning signs of serious health problems.
- ▭ Don't overdress. There is no benefit to excessive sweating and it can even be dangerous.
- ▭ Read about fitness and exercise.
- ▭ Talk about good fitness habits with persons who stay fit.
- ▭ The first step is the hardest, but also the most important. Get up and start!

Four Popular Physical Activities to Consider

Walking - Walking is the most popular form of physical activity. If done on a regular basis, walking can not only help you to lose weight, but will relax you as well. There are some other advantages to walking: It can be done anywhere and anytime; it's free; you already know how to do it; and it can be done by almost anyone. Body posture is important to make your walking as efficient as possible. Keep these pointers in mind when walking.

- ▭ Hold your head erect.
- ▭ Keep your back straight
- ▭ Point your toes straight ahead.
- ▭ Keep your abdomen flat.
- ▭ Swing your arms loosely at your sides.
- ▭ Land on your heel and roll forward off the ball of your foot.
- ▭ Wear shoes that are cushioned and provide support.
- ▭ If you become breathless, you're walking too fast.
- ▭ Don't compete with others - you're not in a race.
- ▭ Make your walk a pleasant experience.

Jogging- Jogging is perhaps the most ideal fitness activity to improve our overall fitness level. People who are unaccustomed to exercise can, with proper progression, advance from being walkers, to walk joggers (woggers), to joggers with little difficulty. Correct posture, pace, number of times you jog per week, and wearing the proper attire are all factors in its effectiveness.

Swimming - Swimming has long been a popular exercise for people who suffer from orthopedic problems or obesity because it reduces pressure on muscles and bones. Swimming has been found to produce relaxation and sound sleep patterns. In comparing swimming to jogging, we can say that 100 yds. of swimming is roughly equivalent to 400 yds. of jogging.

Bicycling - is a good exercise to do with others and is a method of transportation as well. It provides wonderful conditioning for the legs and can improve cardiovascular fitness. Safety precautions are important when bicycling outdoors. (Make sure you wear a bicycle helmet). To improve cardiovascular fitness, cycling should be done at least three times a week for 40-60 minutes each time. A stationary bicycle that has a resistance adjuster is good for regular exercise. It's certainly convenient since you can read or watch TV while you pedal away and the weather doesn't interfere with your exercising.

Nutrition - Eating for Life

The old saying, "You are what you eat" seems to be more true now than ever before. Eating right plays a pivotal role in good health and in disease prevention. The foods you "chews" can help lower your risk for heart disease, stroke, diabetes, osteoporosis, and certain cancers. Do yourself a favor: Eat well to feel well and be well!

The United States Department of Agriculture (U.S.D.A.) and Department of Health and Human Services (HHS) have stated what defines eating well. They call it "Dietary Guidelines for Americans."

These guidelines cover the most up-to-date advice from nutrition scientists and are the basis of federal nutrition policy.

Dietary Guidelines for Americans

- Eat a variety of foods. To make sure you get all of the nutrients and other substances needed for health, choose the recommended number of daily servings from each of the five major food groups displayed in the Food Guide Pyramid. (See the Food Guide Pyramid on page 44.) Vary your choices from each of the food groups.

- Balance the food you eat with physical activity – maintain or improve your weight. Many Americans gain weight in adulthood, increasing their risk for high blood pressure, heart disease, stroke, diabetes, certain types of cancer, arthritis, breathing problems, and other illness. Therefore, most adults should not gain weight. If you are overweight and have one of these problems, you should try to lose weight, or at the very least, not gain weight.

- Choose a diet with plenty of grain products, vegetables, and fruits. These foods provide vitamins, minerals, complex carbohydrates (starch and dietary fiber), and other substances that are important for good health. They are also generally low in fat, depending on how they are prepared and what is added to them at the table.

- Choose a diet low in fat, saturated fat, and cholesterol. High levels of saturated fat and cholesterol in the diet are linked to increased blood cholesterol levels and a greater risk for heart disease. Also fat contains over twice the calories of an equal amount of carbohydrates or protein. A diet low in fat can help you maintain a healthy weight.

- Choose a diet moderate in sugars. Because maintaining a nutritious diet and a healthy weight is very important, sugars should be used in moderation by most healthy people and sparingly by people with low calorie needs. Avoid eating sugars in large amounts and frequent snacks of food and beverages containing sugars that supply unnecessary calories and few nutrients.

- Choose a diet moderate in salt and sodium. A high sodium intake is associated with higher blood pressure. Most evidence suggests that many people at risk for high blood pressure reduce their chances of developing this condition by consuming less salt or sodium.

- If you drink alcoholic beverages, do so in moderation. Moderation is defined as no more than one drink per day for women and no more than two drinks per day for men. When you drink alcoholic beverages in moderation, do so with meals, and when consumption does not put you or others at risk.

What is the Food Guide Pyramid?

An easy way to follow the Dietary Guidelines for Americans is to choose foods daily, using the Food Guide Pyramid. The pyramids of Egypt have withstood the passage of time. Likewise, the Food Guide Pyramid can be used throughout a lifetime as a good foundation of what Americans should eat every day. It is not a rigid prescription, but a general guide that lets you choose a healthful diet that's right for you and members of your family.

The pyramid calls for eating a variety of foods from each group to get the nutrients you need. At the same time, you can get the right amount of calories (and grams of fat) you need to lose or gain weight or maintain a healthy weight by adjusting the number of servings you eat from each group.

> **KEY**
> ◨ Fat (naturally occurring and added)   ◸ Sugars (added)
> These symbols show that fat and added sugars come mostly from fats, oils, and sweets, but can be part of or added to foods from the other food groups as well.

Fats, Oils, & Sweets
USE SPARINGLY

Milk, Yogurt, & Cheese Group
2-3 SERVINGS

Meat, Poultry, Fish, Dry Beans, Eggs, & Nuts Group
2-3 SERVINGS

Vegetable Group
3-5 SERVINGS

Fruit Group
2-4 SERVINGS

Bread, Cereal, Rice, & Pasta Group
6-11 SERVINGS

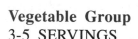

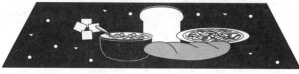
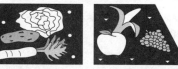

What Counts as a Serving?

▭ Bread, Cereal, Rice and Pasta Group
  - 1 slice of bread
  - 1 ounce of ready-to-eat cereal
  - 1/2 cup of cooked cereal, rice or pasta

▭ Vegetable Group
  - 1 cup of raw, leafy vegetables
  - 1/2 cup of other vegetables, cooked chopped raw
  - 3/4 cup of vegetable juice

▭ Meat, Poultry, Fish, Dry Beans, Eggs and Nuts Group
  - 2-3 ounces of cooked, lean meat, poultry or fish
  - 1/2 cup of cooked dry beans, 1 egg, or 2 tablespoons of peanut butter count as 1 ounce of lean meat

▭ Fruit Group
  - 1 medium apple, banana or orange
  - 1/2 cup of chopped, cooked or canned fruit
  - 3/4 cup of fruit juice

▭ Milk, Yogurt and Cheese Group
  - 1 cup of milk or yogurt
  - 1-1/2 ounces of natural cheese
  - 2 ounces of processed cheese

FYI - Key Nutrition Issues

Balance is the key. Know what to say yes to, what to moderate, and what to go easy on. Say yes to five or more servings of fruits and vegetables a day to get vitamins, minerals, dietary fiber and anti-cancer substances.

Say yes to dietary fiber

Dietary fiber comes from plant foods only. (The part that goes undigested and unabsorbed). Animal foods have no fiber. Aim to get between 20-35 grams of dietary fiber per day. Food labels list the grams of dietary fiber per serving. Read them.

Say yes to calcium

Why? It is needed to strengthen bones and teeth, to help guard against osteoporosis, and to help your heart beat, your blood clot, your muscles flex and your nerves react. Health experts recommend between 800-1500 milligrams of calcium a day for adults. Good food sources are:

- Milk, yogurt, cheese (choose non-fat and low-fat ones).
- Broccoli, collard greens, kale, spinach.
- Legumes, dried beans and peas.
- Tofu (if calcium is used in processing).
- Salmon, sardines (with bones).
- Calcium fortified juices, cereals, breads, etc.

Use sugar, salt, sodium and alcohol in moderation

- Sugar - Many foods that contain large amounts supply calories, are limited in nutrients, and can contribute to tooth decay.
- Salt and Sodium - Most Americans eat more salt and sodium than they need. (Salt contains 40% sodium, 60% chloride). The recommended amount of sodium is between 2400 and 3000 milligrams per day.
- Alcohol - Moderate use means no more than 1-2 drinks per day. 1 per day for women, 2 per day for men. 1 drink = 12 oz. regular beer, 4-5 oz. wine, 1-1/2 oz. distilled spirits (80 proof).

[Note: Women who are trying to conceive or are pregnant should not drink alcoholic beverages.]

Say no to too much fat

Why? Populations with diets high in fat have more obesity and certain types of cancer (breast, colon, prostate). How much is too much? It is recommended that you get less than 30% of total calories from fat.

To figure out how to get less than 30% of calories from fat:

- Take 30% of total calories.
  Example: .30 x 1200 calories = 360 calories.
- Divide the answer by 9 calories/gram (fat contains 9 calories per gram) to get the upper limit of grams of fat per day.
  Example: 360 calories ÷ 9 calories/gram of fat = 40 grams of fat.

For this many Calories	Max. Grams of Fat / Day		
	30% of Calories	25% of Calories	20% of Calories
1200	40 grams	34 grams	28 grams
1500	50 grams	42 grams	34 grams
1800	60 grams	50 grams	40 grams
2000	67 grams	56 grams	44 grams

Read food labels to find out how many grams of fat per serving a food item contains.

Say no to saturated fat

Why? Saturated fat raises blood cholesterol more than anything else in the diet. Saturated fats are generally solid at room temperature. Examples of foods that are high in saturated fat:

- Coconut oil.
- Palm oil.
- Animal fats.
- Dairy foods with fats.
- Cocoa butter.

Say no to too much dietary cholesterol

Why? Dietary cholesterol in excess can contribute to hardening of the arteries.

About cholesterol

Cholesterol is an odorless, white, waxy substance. Cholesterol is made only by animals. It is present in every cell in all parts of the body, including the brain and nervous system, muscle, skin, liver, intestines, heart, and skeleton. There are two sources of cholesterol: The cholesterol our body makes (mostly in the liver) and the cholesterol that is found in animal foods (dietary cholesterol). Examples of foods with cholesterol are:

- Organ meats, such as liver and kidneys.
- Eggs yolks.
- Meats, poultry and fish.
- Fats in dairy products.

Plant foods have no cholesterol.

It is recommended that we do not eat more than 300 milligrams of dietary cholesterol per day.

Your blood cholesterol can be measured using a blood sample taken from your finger or arm. The U.S. government has established the following guidelines for individuals:

Total blood cholesterol

Less than 200 mg/dl .... Desirable
200-239 mg/d .... Borderline High
More than 240 mg/dl .... High

A fasting blood test is not needed to measure total blood cholesterol. Your doctor will probably order a fasting blood test, however, if your total blood cholesterol is elevated. A fasting blood test will reveal a more complete "cholesterol profile." It will give measurements of types of lipoproteins, "packages" in which cholesterol travels in the blood. Two types of lipoproteins of interest are:

Low-density lipoproteins (LDL) - carry most of the cholesterol in the blood. LDL's deposit cholesterol in the artery walls. They are called "bad cholesterol."

High density lipoproteins (HDL) - contain a small amount of cholesterol. HDL's help remove cholesterol from the blood. They are called "good cholesterol."

LDL and HDL cholesterol levels (from a fasting blood test) give a better picture of your risk for coronary heart disease than total cholesterol alone. A **high** LDL-cholesterol and/or a **low** HDL-cholesterol level increases your risk. The following guidelines are used today:

LDL cholesterol

Less than 130 mg/dl .... Desirable
130-159 mg/d .... Borderline High
More than 160 mg/dl .... High

HDL cholesterol

Less than 35 mg/dl .... High Risk
More than 55 mg/dl .... Low Risk

Some health care experts use a ratio of total cholesterol divided by HDL cholesterol to determine risk for heart disease as follows:

Total cholesterol / HDL (ratio)

More than 6.0 .... High Risk
Less than 4.0 .... Low Risk

About triglycerides

Triglycerides are fat-like substances carried through the bloodstream to the tissues. The bulk of the body's fat tissue is in the form of triglycerides, stored for later use as energy. We get triglycerides from the fat in our foods, both animal and plant sources. Normal fasting blood triglyceride levels range from 40-160 mg/dl. They are thought to be elevated if fasting levels are over 250 mg/dl. To lower elevated triglycerides, do the following:

- Lose weight if you are overweight.
- Eat a low-fat diet.
- Limit alcohol.
- Limit sugar and foods with sugar.
- Exercise regularly.

[Note: Some people may need medicine to help lower cholesterol and/or triglycerides in addition to dietary measures. Check with your doctor.]

Weight Control
"Chewsing" Well

Millions of Americans are caught up in the daily struggle to shed unwanted pounds. The link between obesity and such medical conditions as diabetes, high blood pressure and heart disease has been well established. These threats to our health, however, don't always provide the incentives we need to change.

Only a small percent of Americans who try to lose weight seem to keep it off long term. It is not easy to change old habits. Liquid potions, diet pills, powders, crash or fad diets do not prove successful over the long run and can even be harmful.

The three key ingredients for successful weight loss are:
- Regular, physical activity.
- Reduction of caloric intake, especially from fat.
- Modification of eating and exercise behaviors.

What should you do?
- See page 41 to set up a regular exercise program.
- Follow USDA Dietary Guidelines for Americans. (See page 43).

Use the Food Guide Pyramid, but opt for choices in each level that are low in fat (ones inside the pyramid). Limit choices outside the pyramid.

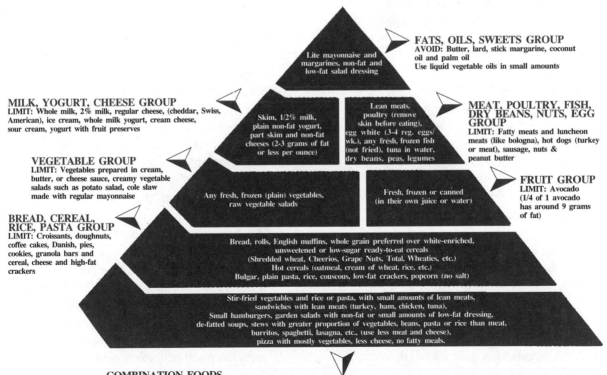

FATS, OILS, SWEETS GROUP
AVOID: Butter, lard, stick margarine, coconut oil and palm oil
Use liquid vegetable oils in small amounts

Lite mayonnaise and margarines, non-fat and low-fat salad dressing

MILK, YOGURT, CHEESE GROUP
LIMIT: Whole milk, 2% milk, regular cheese, (cheddar, Swiss, American), ice cream, whole milk yogurt, cream cheese, sour cream, yogurt with fruit preserves

Skim, 1/2% milk, plain non-fat yogurt, part skim and non-fat cheeses (2-3 grams of fat or less per ounce)

Lean meats, poultry (remove skin before eating), egg white (3-4 reg. eggs/wk.), any fresh, frozen fish (not fried), tuna in water, dry beans, peas, legumes

MEAT, POULTRY, FISH, DRY BEANS, NUTS, EGG GROUP
LIMIT: Fatty meats and luncheon meats (like bologna), hot dogs (turkey or meat), sausage, nuts & peanut butter

VEGETABLE GROUP
LIMIT: Vegetables prepared in cream, butter, or cheese sauce, creamy vegetable salads such as potato salad, cole slaw made with regular mayonnaise

Any fresh, frozen (plain) vegetables, raw vegetable salads

Fresh, frozen or canned (in their own juice or water)

FRUIT GROUP
LIMIT: Avocado (1/4 of 1 avocado has around 9 grams of fat)

BREAD, CEREAL, RICE, PASTA GROUP
LIMIT: Croissants, doughnuts, coffee cakes, Danish, pies, cookies, granola bars and cereal, cheese and high-fat crackers

Bread, rolls, English muffins, whole grain preferred over white-enriched, unsweetened or low-sugar ready-to-eat cereals (Shredded wheat, Cheerios, Grape Nuts, Total, Wheaties, etc.)
Hot cereals (oatmeal, cream of wheat, rice, etc.)
Bulgar, plain pasta, rice, couscous, low-fat crackers, popcorn (no salt)

Stir-fried vegetables and rice or pasta, with small amounts of lean meats, sandwiches with lean meats (turkey, ham, chicken, tuna), Small hamburgers, garden salads with non-fat or small amounts of low-fat dressing, de-fatted soups, stews with greater proportion of vegetables, beans, pasta or rice than meat, burritos, spaghetti, lasagna, etc., (use less meat and cheese), pizza with mostly vegetables, less cheese, no fatty meals.

COMBINATION FOODS
LIMIT: Fried meat and fish sandwiches. Large double decker hamburgers, cheeseburgers, taco salad, hot dogs, Coney Island hot dogs, nachos with cheese, pizza with double cheese and high fat meats like pepperoni and sausage.

Follow Behavior Modification Techniques for Weight Control

Use the suggestions below to change the way you eat.

Eating Pace

▢ Eat slowly. Chances are you will eat less.

▢ Chew and swallow each bite thoroughly before beginning another.

▢ Take sips of water between bites.

Eating Mood

▢ Make a point to eat only when relaxed. (Many people eat to reduce tension).

▢ Instead of thinking of "not eating," think of showing respect for your body by refusing to overeat.

▢ Concentrate on feelings of being bloated or stuffed before you overeat. Be aware of these negative physical sensations. This will help you limit your food intake.

Eating Out

▢ Choose restaurants where a variety of low-fat foods are available. Decide what you'll eat ahead of time.

▢ Don't starve yourself all day prior to dining out.

▢ Avoid "All-you-can-eat" restaurants.

▢ Consider ordering "a la carte" or "half orders" to keep portions small.

Eating With Others

▢ Beware of "Saboteurs" who try to undermine your weight loss efforts. They may feel threatened by your success.

▢ Tell others about your long term weight loss goals.

▢ Meet friends for a walk instead of lunch.

Self Rewards

▢ Spend some time imagining yourself at your healthy body weight. Visualize in detail how you look, feel and think as the healthier you.

▢ Give yourself positive reinforcement each day you follow your eating plan. Choose something that's a little special like a stroll in the park, a long distance call, some "me-time."

▢ Keep saying positive self statements to yourself or in front of a mirror. Say "I am in control" or "I choose to respect myself." This will go a long way when you find yourself wanting to eat at inappropriate times.

Miscellaneous Techniques

▢ Know the difference between appetite and hunger. Appetite is a psychological desire for food, while hunger is a true physical need for it.

▢ Use smaller-sized plates for meals.

▢ To avoid impulse buying, shop only from a well planned list and never shop when hungry.

▢ Blast out your desire for food by yelling the word "STOP."

▢ Plan your snacks in advance.

▢ Put on tight clothes if you feel a desire to binge.

▢ Don't eat just because others are. Wait until you are really hungry.

▢ Above all, maintain a positive attitude. Commit to being a positive thinker. Focus on what you can do and what rewards come from eating well and exercising. They will result in improved health, a better mental attitude, more energy and improved appearance and performance, etc.

Alcohol - Use Without Abuse

The effects of alcohol vary from person to person. The following factors influence the intoxication properties of alcohol:

- Amount of food already in the stomach.
- Presence of other medications already in the system.
- Pace that drinks are consumed.
- The person's mental/emotional condition.
- The individual's tolerance level.
- An individual's body weight.

The Effects of Alcohol

There is a relationship between the blood alcohol concentration in our system and how we are affected by it. The chart below describes what we can expect to see as more and more alcohol is consumed.

Amount of Distilled Spirit Consumed in 2 hours (ounces)	Alcohol In Blood (percent)	Typical Effects (varies per individual)
3	0.05	Loosening of judgment, thought, and restraint. Release of tension; carefree sensation.
4.5	0.08	Tensions and inhibitions of everyday life lessened.
6	0.10	Voluntary motor action affected; hand and arm movements, walk and speech clumsy.
10	0.20	Severe impairment, staggering, loud, incoherent, emotionally unstable, very drunk; 100 times greater risk of traffic accident.
14	0.30	Deeper areas of brain affected. Parts affecting stimulus response and understanding confused, stuporous.
18	0.40	Asleep, difficult to arouse, incapable of voluntary action, equivalent of surgical anesthesia.
22	0.50	Coma, anesthesia of centers controlling breathing and heartbeat. Death.

Know Your Limit[1]

Body Weight	# of Drinks[2] during a 2 hour period									
100 lbs.	1	2	3	4	5	6	7	8	9	10
120	1	2	3	4	5	6	7	8	9	10
140	1	2	3	4	5	6	7	8	9	10
160	1	2	3	4	5	6	7	8	9	10
180	1	2	3	4	5	6	7	8	9	10
200	1	2	3	4	5	6	7	8	9	10
220	1	2	3	4	5	6	7	8	9	10
240	1	2	3	4	5	6	7	8	9	10

Be Careful Driving BAC* to .05	Driving May Be Impaired BAC .05-.09[3]	Do Not Drive BAC .10 and up

[1] This chart provides averages only. Individuals may vary, and factors such as food in the stomach, medication and fatigue can affect your tolerance.

[2] One drink is 1-1/4 oz. of 80 proof liquor, 12 oz. of beer or 4 oz. of wine.

[3] The BAC percentages for impairment and intoxication vary from state to state.

* BAC = Blood Alcohol Content

Developed by Techniques for Alcohol Management. Used with permission.

If you're in doubt about your ability to drive, play it safe. Don't drive!

Preventing Alcohol Problems

Below are some guidelines to follow to prevent the onset of problems due to alcohol.

- ☐ Be aware of the blood alcohol concentration danger levels.
- ☐ Don't develop a routine of social drinking or a pattern of drinking at a particular time of the day.
- ☐ Eat some food along with a drink and never start to drink on an empty stomach.
- ☐ Avoid social pressures to drink. Be assertive in your choice not to drink. Remember, parties are for socializing, not to get intoxicated.
- ☐ Get help if you suspect an alcohol dependency problem. Don't wait until the problem worsens.
- ☐ Remember, an entire family suffers when a member has an untreated alcohol problem.
- ☐ Check with your doctor about drinking alcohol while taking prescription and over-the-counter medication.
- ☐ Don't drive if you've been drinking and don't be a passenger of someone who has been drinking.
- ☐ If you have a drink, drink it slowly. Never gulp it down due to thirst. If thirsty, drink water first.
- ☐ Pregnant women should avoid alcohol.
- ☐ Skip that offer of "one for the road."
- ☐ Be wary of unfamiliar drinks and choose not to consume them.

Be aware that nothing will sober you up but time. Your liver will only metabolize about one ounce of alcohol per hour.

Playing it Safe - Tips for Home

Most accidents happen at home. If you think your house is "home, safe home," take a look around. At first glance it may look orderly, but certain trouble spots can lead to cuts, falls, burns, or other injuries. The following room-by-room checklist can alert you to accidents waiting to happen.

Kitchen

- ☐ Cleaners and dangerous chemicals should be stored out of children's reach.
- ☐ Scissors, knives, ice picks, and other sharp tools should be stored separately from other utensils and out of the reach of children.
- ☐ Towels, curtains, and other flammable materials should hang a safe distance from heat sources like the stove.
- ☐ Kitchen fans and stove ventilation exhausts should be clean and in good working order.
- ☐ Electrical cords should run a safe distance from the sink or range.
- ☐ Electrical outlets should not be overloaded.
- ☐ A sturdy step stool should be available to help reach high cabinets.
- ☐ Vinyl floors should be cleaned with nonskid wax.
- ☐ A nonskid floor mat should be in place in front of the sink.
- ☐ The kitchen should be well-lit.

Bedroom

- ☐ Electrical cords should be in good working order and tucked away from foot traffic.
- ☐ Electrical outlets should not be overloaded.
- ☐ Electric blankets should not be covered by bedspreads or other blankets when in use.
- ☐ Carpeting should be secured to the floor.
- ☐ A night-light should be put between the bed and the bathroom or hallway.
- ☐ The bedroom telephone should be easy to reach, even from the floor, if necessary.

- Ashtrays, irons, electric hair curlers, and other potential fire hazards should be located away from bedding, curtains, or other flammable material.
- Smoke detectors should be located near entrances to rooms, and their batteries should be checked often and replaced when needed.

Bathroom

- Floor mats should have non-skid backing.
- Rubber mats or adhesive-backed strips should be in place in the bathtub or shower stall.
- A support bar should be securely installed in the bathtub or shower stall.
- Hair dryers, electric shavers, or other electric appliances should be kept away from water and unplugged when not in use.
- A light switch should be located near the bathroom entrance or entrances.

Halls and Stairs

- Halls and stairs should be well-lit, with a light switch at each end of a stairway.
- If a staircase is dimly lit, the top and bottom steps should be marked with reflective tape.
- Sturdy hand rails should be securely installed on both sides of each stairway.
- Floor covering on stairs and in halls should be skid-proof or carpeted and not creased or frayed.
- Stairways should be clear of shoes, books, toys, tools, or other clutter.
- When young children are in the house, gates should block access to stairways.

Basement and Garage

- To avoid confusion and misuse, all chemicals and cleaners should be kept in their original containers and out of children's reach.
- Hazardous chemicals should be kept under lock and key and out of children's reach.
- Sharp or otherwise potentially hazardous tools should be in good working order and kept off limits to children.
- Gasoline and other flammable materials should be stored in airtight containers and away from heat sources (outside the home, if possible).
- Buy a radon test kit from your state department of health or department of environmental protection, or contact the Environmental Control Agency, 230 South Dearborn Street, Chicago, IL 60604 for information on radon testing. (Radon is an invisible gas that causes health problems if it builds up in homes and can't escape). If your home has high radon levels, hire a reliable radon expert to help you reduce levels of this gas in your home.

Elsewhere around the House

- Outdoor porches and walkways should be kept clear of ice in winter weather.
- Window screens should be securely fastened, especially if small children are around.
- Do not have poisonous plants in your yard or inside your house.
- Do not leave children unattended near swimming pools and playground equipment.
- Plan escape routes in case of fire or other emergencies. Talk about these with household members and practice using them.

Take steps to remedy unsafe situations as soon as possible.

Pregnancy - Planning a Healthy Baby

Healthy moms have healthy babies. If you plan to, or become pregnant, take the following steps to be sure your pregnancy is a healthy one and that your baby gets off to a good start.

- Consider genetic tests or counseling if you or your husband have a family history of genetic disorders, if you are 35 or older or if your husband is 60 or older.
- Have a complete medical exam, including a gynecological exam. A number of medical conditions can jeopardize the health of mother and child:
  - Obesity.
  - High blood pressure.
  - Diabetes.
  - German measles (Rubella).
  - RH negative blood factor (after the first pregnancy).
  - Sexually transmitted disease (STDs) and AIDS or having the AIDS virus (HIV).
- Take measures to control and/or treat all medical conditions and take care of your health before you get pregnant and when you are pregnant. If you have a chronic medical condition, ask your doctor how it may affect your pregnancy.
- Consult your doctor before taking any medication.
- Start prenatal vitamins while trying to get pregnant. This may prevent certain birth defects, such as neural tube defects like spina bifida. Continue to take vitamin-mineral supplements as prescribed by your doctor throughout your pregnancy.
- Ask your doctor or a dietitian to outline a meal plan that meets the special nutritional needs created by pregnancy.

- Avoid alcohol, nicotine and illicit drugs, as they can harm you and your unborn baby.
- Limit your intake of caffeine each day to no more than that contained in 2-3 cups of coffee, or about 400 milligrams.
- Follow your doctor's advice about weight gain. The amount of weight you gain should depend on your pre-pregnancy weight and health status, as well as your ethnic background. If you're markedly overweight, plan to lose excess pounds before becoming pregnant.
- Exercise in moderation, three times a week with your doctor's okay. Some activities considered safe during pregnancy are walking, golf, swimming, bicycling and low impact aerobics.
- Practice relaxation and other stress control techniques. Doctors think emotional stress may constrict the blood supply to the uterus and placenta, the baby's sole source of oxygen and nutrients.
- Enroll in childbirth preparation classes.
- If you own a cat, arrange for someone else to empty the litter box. Cat excrement can transmit a disease called toxoplasmosis. If you're infected while pregnant, your baby may be stillborn, born prematurely or suffer serious damage to the brain, eyes or other parts of the body. It is safe, however, to handle or pet the cat.
- Be informed. Know the warning signs of pregnancy complications. These include increasing blood pressure and early labor. Getting treatment early is important.

Preventing Preterm Labor

A pregnant woman who starts to have her baby too soon is in preterm labor. A full-term pregnancy is about 40 weeks. Babies born before 37 weeks are considered preterm and may have health problems because they were born early.

The cause of preterm labor is not completely understood. Any pregnant woman can have preterm labor. The following conditions are associated with an increased risk of having a preterm baby:

☐ Previous preterm birth.

☐ Three or more miscarriages in a row.

☐ Bleeding problems.

☐ Pregnant with more than one baby.

☐ Abnormally shaped uterus.

☐ Daughter of a mother who took DES (a medication used from the 1940s to 1970s by pregnant women to prevent miscarriage).

☐ Infections of the urinary tract, vagina, cervix, etc.

☐ Not enough weight gain, poor diet, lack of prenatal care.

☐ Smoking, drinking alcohol, misusing drugs.

☐ Severe emotional stress.

☐ Mother is younger than 18 or older than 35.

This is not an all-inclusive list. If you have questions about these conditions, discuss them with your doctor.

Being at an increased risk does not mean a woman will have a preterm baby. Whether you are at risk or not, learn the warning signs and how to feel your uterus (womb) to tell if you are in labor. It is possible to prevent a baby from being born too early, in some cases, if early warning signs are recognized and steps are taken to stop labor.

The following are warning signs of preterm labor:

☐ Contractions come every 15 minutes or closer and last from 20 seconds to 2 minutes each.

☐ Contractions come closer together as time goes on.

☐ Menstrual-like cramps come and go or don't go away.

☐ Pressure in your pelvis, back, or insides of your thighs. It feels like the baby is pushing down.

☐ Dull backache below your waist comes and goes or doesn't go away.

☐ Change in vaginal discharge.

☐ Fluid leaking from the vagina.

☐ A strange feeling that something is not right.

☐ Fever of 100.4°F or higher and/or chills.

Remember that preterm labor is usually not painful. If you have any of the signs of preterm labor, do the following:

☐ Lie down, tilted toward your left side for 1 hour. Do not lie flat on your back.

☐ Drink 2 to 3 glasses of water or juice during this hour.

☐ Keep feeling your stomach for uterine contractions. Time your contractions.

If the signs do not go away in 1 hour, or if you have fluid leaking from your vagina, do not wait. Call your health care provider! When you call, tell your nurse or doctor:

☐ Your name.

☐ When your baby is due.

☐ What signs you are having.

☐ How often you are having contractions.

SECTION II
Common Health Problems

Introduction

Getting sick costs more than ever before. All these health care costs are going up:

- Insurance Rates.
- Co-pays.
- Deductibles.
- Tests.
- Prescriptions.
- Doctor office and health clinic visits.

You have to make a lot of decisions when you get sick, such as:

- Should I go to the emergency room?
- Should I call my doctor?
- Can I wait and see if it gets better?
- Can I take care of it myself?
- What self treatments should I do?

This section of HealthySelf can help you. It presents 75 common health problems and tells what you can do when you have one of them.

Sometimes you can treat these problems with self-care. Sometimes you need medical help. HealthySelf can help you ask the right questions and find the answers to take care of your health.

Each health problem is divided into 3 parts:

- Facts about the problem: What it is, what causes it, symptoms and treatments.
- YES or NO questions to help you decide if you should get help fast, call your doctor, see your doctor or provide self-care.
- A list of self-care treatments for the problem.

How to Use This Section

- Find the problem in the Table of Contents in the beginning of the book and go to that page. The problems are listed in alphabetical order.
- Read about the problem, what causes it (if known), it's symptoms and treatments.
- Ask yourself the "Questions to Ask." Start at the top of the flow chart and answer YES or NO to each question. Follow the arrows until you get to one of these answers:
  - Seek Emergency Care.
  - See Doctor.
  - Call Doctor.
  - Use Self-Care.

What the Instructions Mean

Seek Emergency Care

You should get help fast. Go to the hospital emergency room or call for emergency medical service (EMS) from your city EMS department or local ambulance service.

You may not need a hospital emergency room or EMS services for some emergencies if they do not threaten life or can be taken care of at out-patient centers. An example is a sprained ankle. Ask your doctor ahead of time where you should go for a sprained ankle or similar type of problem that needs prompt care but not necessarily emergency care. Some hospital emergency departments may have "Prompt Care" areas to treat minor injuries or illnesses.

Make sure you know a phone number for emergency medical help. Write it down near your phone and in the "Emergency Phone Numbers" listed on page 1 of this book.

See Doctor

The term "Doctor" can be used for a number of health care providers. They include:

- Your physician.
- Your Health Maintenance Organization (HMO) clinic, primary doctor or other designated health professional.
- Walk-in clinic or urgent care center.
- Physician's assistants (P.A.s), Certified Nurses (C.N.s), who work with your doctor.
- Home health care provider.
- Your dentist.

When you see the "See Doctor" symbol, you should do so as soon as you can. You may need medicine or treatment to keep the problem from getting worse. Call first and ask for an appointment or for immediate care. Tell the nurse or receptionist what's wrong if you can't talk to your doctor directly. If you can't be seen soon, ask for a referral. A referral from your doctor can help you get to see someone else who can help you.

Call Doctor

Call your doctor and state the problem. He/she can decide what you should do. He/she may:

- Tell you to make an appointment to be seen.
- Send you to a laboratory for tests.
- Prescribe medicine or treatment over the phone.
- Give you specific instructions to treat the problem.

Use Self-Care

You can probably take care of the problems yourself if you answered NO to all the questions. Use the Self-Care Tips that are listed. But call your doctor if you don't feel better soon. You may have some other problem.

chapter 10

EYES, EARS, NOSE & THROAT

Earaches

Earaches can be mild or very painful. They are a sign that something is wrong. The most common cause of an earache is plugged eustachian tubes. These tubes go from the back of the throat to your middle ear. When the eustachian tube gets blocked, fluid gathers, causing pain. Things that make this happen include an infection of the middle ear, colds, sinus infections, and allergies. Other things that can cause ear pain include changes in air pressure in a plane, something stuck in the ear, too much ear wax, tooth problems, and ear injuries.

Very bad ear pain should be treated by a doctor. Treatment will depend on its cause. Most often this includes pain relievers, an antibiotic for infection and methods to dry up or clear the blocked ear canal. You can, however, use self-care tips if ear pain is mild and produces no other symptoms. One example is with a <u>mild</u> case of "swimmers ear" which affects the outer ear. (See Self-Care Tips on page 57).

Prevention

Much can be done to prevent earaches. Heed the old saying, "Never put anything smaller than your elbow into your ear". This includes cotton-tipped swabs, bobby pins, your fingers, etc. Doing so could damage your eardrum. When you blow your nose, do so gently, one nostril at a time. Don't smoke. Smoking and second hand smoke can increase the risk of infection.

Questions to Ask

Has the pain occurred as a result of a blow to the ear or recent head trauma?

NO

flowchart continued in next column

Are the following symptoms present with the earache?
- **Stiff neck**
- **Fever**
- **Drowsiness**
- **Nausea, vomiting**

YES →

NO

Are there any of the following signs of infection?
- **Fever (especially 102°F or higher)**
- **Sticky, green, or bloody discharge**
- **Severe ear pain and/or increased pain when wiggling the ear lobe**

YES →

NO

Is the earache persistent and more than mild and occurring after the following?
- **A mild ear injury**
- **Blowing your nose hard or many times**
- **Sticking an object of any kind in the ear**
- **A cold, sinus, or upper respiratory infection**
- **Swimming, and is it extremely painful when the earlobe is wiggled or touched**
- **Exposure to extremely loud noises (Examples: Rock concerts, heavy machinery)**

YES →

NO

Is the earache accompanied by hearing loss, ringing in the ears, dizziness or nausea?

YES →

NO

flowchart continued on next page

Earaches, continued

Are any of the following signs and symptoms present in an infant or small child, especially following an upper respiratory infection, a cold, air travel, or in a child with a history of ear problems?
- **Constant pulling, touching, or tugging at one or both ears**
- **Fever**
- **Constant crying despite being comforted**
- **Ear or ears that are hot and sensitive to the touch**
- **Unresponsiveness or excessive sensitivity to loud noises, a bell, or to the sound of your voice**
- **Irritability and sleeplessness, especially at night or when lying down**

YES SEE DOCTOR

NO

Has a small object been stuck in the ear that cannot be easily removed or has an insect gotten in the ear that cannot safely be removed?

YES SEE DOCTOR

NO

Does the earache occur with jaw pain, headache, and a clicking sound when opening and closing the mouth?

YES CALL DOCTOR

NO

 USE SELF-CARE

Self-Care Tips

To reduce pain:
- ☐ Place a warm washcloth or heating pad (set on low, adults only) next to the ear. Some health professionals recommend putting an ice bag or ice in a wet washcloth over the painful ear for 20 minutes.

- ☐ Take acetaminophen, aspirin, ibuprofen, or naproxen sodium. *[Note: Do not give aspirin or any medication containing salicylates to anyone 19 years of age or younger, unless directed by a physician, due to its association with Reye's Syndrome, a potentially fatal condition.]*

To open up the eustachian tubes and help them drain:
- ☐ Sit up.
- ☐ Prop your head up when you sleep.
- ☐ Yawn. (This helps move the muscles that open the eustachian tubes).
- ☐ Chew gum or suck on hard candy. (This is especially helpful during pressure changes that take place during air travel but can also be useful during the middle of the night if you wake up with ear pain.) (Do not give to children under 5).
- ☐ Stay awake during take-offs and landings when traveling by air.
- ☐ Take an oral decongestant such as Sudafed which can dry up the fluid in the ear that causes the pain. Decongestant nasal sprays can be used, but not for more than three days or as directed by your doctor. Take a decongestant:
  - At the first sign of a cold if you have gotten ear infections often after previous colds.
  - One hour before you land when you travel by air if you have a cold or know your sinuses are going to block up.
- ☐ Take a steamy shower.
- ☐ Use a cool-mist vaporizer, especially at night.
- ☐ Drink plenty of cool water.
- ☐ Gently, but firmly, blow through your nose while holding both nostrils closed until you hear a pop. This will help promote ear drainage. This can be done several times a day.
- ☐ Feed a baby their bottle in an upright position, not lying down.

In treating a mild case of "swimmers ear", the goal is to clean and dry the outer ear canal without doing further damage to the top layer of skin. What you can do:
- ☐ Shake your head to expel trapped water.
- ☐ Dry the ear canal. Take a clean facial tissue. Twist each corner into a tip and gently place each tip into the ear canal for 10 seconds. Repeat with the other ear using a new tissue.

Self-Care Tips continued on next page

Earaches, continued

- Use an over-the-counter product such as Swim-Ear. Drop it into the ears to fight infection. Follow package directions.
- Do not remove ear wax. This coats the ear canal and protects it from moisture.

To avoid getting "swimmer's ear":

- Wear wax or silicone ear plugs that can be softened and shaped to fit your ears. They are available at most drug stores.
- Wear a bathing cap to help keep water from getting into the ears.
- Don't swim in dirty water.
- Swim on the surface of the water instead of underneath the water.

Eye Strain from Computers

Office workers have their share of work-related hazards. People who use video display terminals (VDTs) may often complain of eyestrain, pain, stiffness in their backs and shoulders, and stress. These complaints can be a result of:

- Using a VDT for long time periods.
- Improper positioning of the VDT.
- Poor lighting.
- Poor posture.
- Tight deadlines.

VDT users can protect themselves from the physical problems that go with using them with the Self-Care Tips listed in the next column.

Questions To Ask

Do you still have eye strain, pain and stiffness in back and shoulders despite using Self-Care Tips provided?

Self-Care Tips

To prevent eyestrain:

- Reduce glare. Keep the VDT away from you and at right angles to a window. Turn off or shield overhead lights. Wear a visor to block overhead lights if necessary.
- Place your paperwork close enough that you don't have to keep refocusing when switching from the screen to the paper. Use a paper document holder placed at the same height as the VDT screen.
- Place the screen so that your line of sight is 10 to 15 degrees (about one-third of a 45-degree angle) below horizontal.
- Dust off the screen often.
- Blink often to keep your eyes from getting dry.
- Use "artificial tear" eye drops if needed.
- Tell your eye specialist that you use a VDT. Glasses and contacts worn for other activities may not be good for work on a VDT. (With bifocals, the near vision part of the lens is good for looking down, as when you read, but not straight ahead, as you do when looking at a video display screen. So you may need single-vision lenses for VDT work).
- If the image on the VDT screen is blurred, dull, or flickers, have it serviced right away.
- Try to keep the VDT screen two feet away from your eyes.

To prevent muscle tension when you work on a VDT:

- Use a chair that supports your back and can be easily adjusted to a height that feels right for you.
- Take a 15 minute break if you can, for every 2 hours you use a VDT. Get up and go for a short walk for example.
- Do stretching exercises of the neck, shoulder, and lower back every 1 to 2 hours.
  - Rotate your head in a circular motion, first clockwise, then counterclockwise.
  - Shrug your shoulders up, down, backward, and forward.
  - While standing or sitting, bend at the waist, leaning first to the left, then to the right.

Hay Fever

Despite its name, hay fever has nothing to do with hay or fever. A nineteenth-century physician called it this because he began to sneeze every time he entered a hay barn. But hay fever is, in fact, a reaction of the upper respiratory tract to anything to which you may be allergic. The medical term for hay fever is "allergic rhinitis". Symptoms include itchy, watery eyes, runny, itchy nose, congestion, and sneezing. Hay fever is most common in spring and fall (when ragweed is particularly troublesome), but some people have it all year. You can try to avoid things that give you hay fever. Talk to your doctor if that doesn't help. He or she may prescribe antihistamines, decongestants, and or nasal sprays. Here's what these do:

- Antihistamines stop your body from making histamine, a substance your body makes when you are exposed to an allergen. Histamine causes many allergic symptoms. For best results, take the antihistamine 30 minutes before going outside. *[Note: Some over-the-counter antihistamines may cause more drowsiness than prescription ones. Also, care should be taken when driving and operating machinery since antihistamines can make you drowsy.]*

- Decongestants shrink the blood vessels in your nose. These do not usually cause drowsiness.

- Don't use a nasal spray for more than three days at a time unless directed by your doctor. You may become dependent on it.

It is best to take what your doctor prescribes instead of experimenting with over-the-counter products on your own.

Your doctor may prescribe other things, like Cromolyn sodium or steroids. He or she may suggest allergy shots if your hay fever is very bad. First, you take a skin test. Then you get shots that have a tiny bit of the allergen. The shots help your body get used to the allergen, so it won't be so sensitive.

Questions To Ask

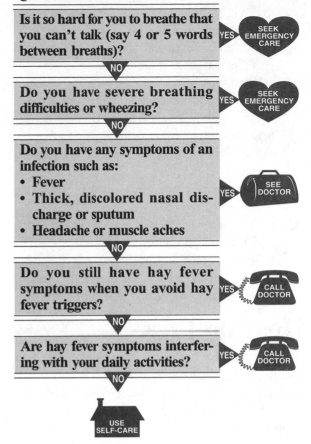

Is it so hard for you to breathe that you can't talk (say 4 or 5 words between breaths)? YES → SEEK EMERGENCY CARE

NO

Do you have severe breathing difficulties or wheezing? YES → SEEK EMERGENCY CARE

NO

Do you have any symptoms of an infection such as:
- **Fever**
- **Thick, discolored nasal discharge or sputum**
- **Headache or muscle aches**

YES → SEE DOCTOR

NO

Do you still have hay fever symptoms when you avoid hay fever triggers? YES → CALL DOCTOR

NO

Are hay fever symptoms interfering with your daily activities? YES → CALL DOCTOR

NO

USE SELF-CARE

Self-Care Tips

Try to stay away from things that give you hay fever:

- Let someone else do outside chores. Mowing the lawn or raking leaves can make you very sick if you are allergic to pollen from grains, trees, or weeds. It's a problem if you are allergic to molds, too.

- Keep windows and doors shut and stay inside when the pollen count or humidity is high. Early morning is sometimes the worst.

- Put an air conditioner or air cleaner in your house, especially in your bedroom. Be sure to clean the filter often.

Self-Care Tips continued on next page

Hay Fever, continued

▭ Try to keep dust, mold, and pollen away from you at home and work:
  - Dust and vacuum your home often. Wear a dust and pollen mask if necessary.
  - Wash rugs.
  - Take carpets and drapes out of your bedroom.
  - Cover your mattress with a plastic cover.
  - Do not use a feather pillow.
  - Stay away from stuffed animals. They collect dust.
  - Don't have pets, or keep your pets outside the house.
  - Don't hang sheets and blankets outside to dry. Pollen can get on them.
  - Shower, bathe and wash your hair following heavy exposure to pollen, dust, etc.

▭ Avoid tobacco smoke and other air pollutants.

Hearing Loss

Do people seem to mumble a lot lately? Do you have trouble hearing in church or theaters? Is it hard to pick up what others say at the dinner table or at family gatherings? Does your family ask you to turn down the volume on the TV or radio?

These are signs of gradual, age-related hearing loss called presbycusis. High pitched sounds are the ones to go first. Hearing loss from presbycusis cannot be restored, but hearing aids, along with the Self-Care Tips listed on page 61 can be helpful.

Hearing loss can also result from other things:

▭ Acoustic trauma - This may be caused by a blow to the ear or from excessive noise. Excessive noise includes that heard from low-flying airplanes when living near an airport, when flying in an airplane, or when working with heavy, loud machinery.

▭ Blood vessel disorders including high blood pressure.

▭ A blood clot that travels to nerves in the ear.

▭ Ear wax that blocks the ear canal.

▭ Chronic middle ear infections, or an infection of the inner ear.

▭ Meniere's disease (a disease marked by excess fluid in canals of the inner ear which help maintain balance).

▭ Multiple sclerosis.

▭ Syphilis.

▭ Brain tumor.

Babies and young children should have their hearing checked during routine office visits. You may notice that your child does not hear properly, however, if he/she does not respond to sounds and is not learning to speak as quickly as you think they should. Children can be born with hearing loss or a hearing impairment or develop hearing loss from an ear or upper respiratory infection.

Questions to Ask

In a child: Does the child not respond to any sound, even a whistle or loud clap? (Did the child's mother have German measles when pregnant with the child)? Does the child not respond to sounds after experiencing any of these things?
- **Recent earache or upper respiratory infection**
- **Airplane travel**

YES

NO

In a child or adult: Do you have any of the following with the hearing loss?
- **Discharge from the ear**
- **Earache**
- **Dizziness or feeling that things are spinning around you**
- **Recent ear or upper respiratory infection**
- **Feeling that the ears are blocked or filled with wax**

YES

NO

flowchart continued on next page

Hearing Loss, continued

Can you <u>not</u> hear a regular (non-digital) watch ticking when held next to the ear? YES	**SEE DOCTOR**

↓ NO

Do you hear a ringing sound in one or both ears all of the time? YES	**SEE DOCTOR**

↓ NO

Did you lose your hearing after being exposed to loud noises such as those associated with airplanes, work or hobby related loud noises (i.e., heavy machinery, power tools, firearms, etc.) and has this not gotten better? YES	**CALL DOCTOR**

↓ NO

USE SELF-CARE

Self-Care Tips

For gradual, age-related hearing loss (presbycusis):
- Ask people to speak clearly, distinctly, and in a normal tone.
- Look at people when they are talking to you. Watch their expressions to help you understand what they are saying. Ask them to face you.
- Try to limit background noise when having a conversation.
- In a church or theater, sit up front.
- To rely on sight instead of sound, install a buzzer, flasher, or amplifier on your telephone, door chime, and alarm clock. Also, an audiologist (hearing therapist) may be able to show you other techniques for "training" yourself to hear better.

To Clear Ear Wax: (Use only if you know that the eardrum is not perforated. Check with your doctor if you are in doubt).
- Lie on your side. Using a syringe or medicine dropper, carefully squeeze a few drops of lukewarm water into your ear (or have someone else do this). Let the water remain there for 10-15 minutes and then shake it out. Do this again,

but use a few drops of hydrogen peroxide, mineral oil or an over-the-counter cleaner such as Murine Ear Drops or Debrox. Let the excess fluid flow out of the ear.
- After several minutes, follow the same procedure using warm water again, letting it remain there for 10-15 minutes. Tilt the head to allow it to drain out of the ear.

You can repeat this entire procedure again in three hours if the ear wax has not cleared.

To prevent hearing loss:
- Don't put cotton-tipped swabs, fingers, bobby pins, etc. in your ear.
- Don't blow your nose with too much force. It is better to do so "gently" with a tissue or handkerchief held loosely over the nostrils.
- Avoid places that have loud noises (airports, construction sites, etc.). Protect your ears with earplugs.
- Keep the volume on "Walkmans", car stereos, etc., on low. If someone else can hear the music when you have earphones on your head, the volume is too loud.
- Follow your doctor's advice for disorders that can cause hearing loss (Example: High blood pressure, Meniere's disease, etc.).
- Avoid prolonged use of medicines that cause hearing loss or overdosing on such medications. (Example: Heavy use of aspirin, streptomycin, quinine).

Also be aware of things that can help you hear sounds if your hearing is impaired.
- Hearing aids (See your doctor).
- Devices made to assist in hearing sounds from the TV and radio.
- Special equipment that can be installed in your telephone by the telephone company.
- Portable devices made especially to amplify sounds. (These can be used for movies, classes, meetings, etc.).

Hiccups

Hiccups are simple enough to explain: Your diaphragm (the major muscle involved in breathing which sits like a cap over the stomach) goes into spasm. Things that promote hiccups are:

- Eating too fast, which causes you to swallow air along with food.
- Eating fatty foods to the point where they make the stomach full enough to irritate the diaphragm.

According to a doctor who studies hiccups, there is a hiccup center in the brain which triggers a spasm of the esophagus setting in motion the cycle leading to hiccups. This, he thinks, is a protective mechanism to keep a person from choking on food or drink. Luckily, hiccups are generally harmless and don't last very long.

Questions To Ask

Do the hiccups occur with severe abdominal pain and spitting up of blood or blood in the stools? **YES** → SEEK EMERGENCY CARE

NO

Have the hiccups lasted longer than 8 hours in an adult or 3 hours in a child? **YES** → CALL DOCTOR

NO

Have the hiccups started only after taking prescription medicine? **YES** → CALL DOCTOR

NO

USE SELF-CARE

Self-Care Tips

Luckily, there's no shortage of hiccup cures, and better still, most of them work (although some baffle medical science). A study reported in the New England Journal of Medicine found that 1 teaspoon of ordinary table sugar, swallowed dry, cured hiccups immediately in 19 out of 20 people. (Some of whom had been hiccuping for as long as six weeks). If this doesn't stop the hiccups right away, repeat it 3 times at 2 minute intervals. *[Note: For young children, use a teaspoon of corn syrup.]*

Other popular folk remedies worth trying include:

- Hold your tongue with your thumb and index finger and gently pull it forward.
- With your neck bent backward, hold your breath for a count of ten. Exhale immediately and drink a glass of water.
- Breathe into and out of a paper (not plastic) bag.
- Swallow a small amount of finely cracked ice.
- Massage the back of the roof of your mouth with a cotton swab. A finger works equally well.
- Eat dry bread slowly.
- Drink a glass of water rapidly.

Laryngitis

Disc jockeys get laryngitis. So do actors, politicians, and others who talk for hours. But ordinary people who overuse their voices get laryngitis, too. Perhaps you cheer too loudly and too often at a basketball game. Or perhaps you lose your voice for no apparent reason.

Air pollution, or spending an evening in a smoky room can also irritate the larynx (voice box) and cause laryngitis. Infections, too, can inflame the larynx. When your larynx is irritated or inflamed, your voice becomes hoarse, husky, and weak. Sometimes laryngitis is painless, but you may get a sore throat, fever or dry cough, a tickling sensation in the back of the throat, or have trouble swallowing. Smoking, drinking alcohol, breathing cold air, and continuing to use already-distressed vocal cords can make the situation worse.

Questions To Ask

Is it hard for you to breathe or swallow or are you coughing up blood? **YES** → SEEK EMERGENCY CARE

NO

Do you have a high fever or are you coughing up blood or yellow-green sputum? **YES** → CALL DOCTOR

NO

flowchart continued on next page

Laryngitis, continued

Do you have hard, swollen lymph glands in your neck or do you feel like you have a "lump in your throat"? YES → CALL DOCTOR

NO ↓

Has the hoarseness lasted more than a week in a child or more than a month in an adult? YES → CALL DOCTOR

NO ↓

Do you have two or more of these problems?
- **Bothered by the cold more than usual**
- **Dry hair or skin**
- **Gaining weight for no reason**
- **Feeling very tired for no reason**

YES → CALL DOCTOR

NO ↓

USE SELF-CARE

Self-Care Tips

- Don't talk if you don't need to. Use a note pad and pencil to write notes instead. If you must speak, do so softly, but don't whisper.
- Use a cool mist humidifier in your home, especially in your bedroom.
- Drink lots of warm drinks. Tea with honey is good.
- Gargle with warm salt water (1/4 teaspoon of salt in 1/2 cup of water).
- Take a hot shower or steam bath.
- Don't smoke. Stay away from places with smoky air.
- Suck on cough drops, throat lozenges or hard candy. (Do not give to children under age 5).
- Take aspirin, acetaminophen, ibuprofen, or naproxen sodium. *[Note: Do not give aspirin or any medication containing salicylates to anyone 19 years of age or younger, unless directed by a physician, due to its association with Reye's Syndrome, a potentially fatal condition.]*

Nosebleeds

Nosebleeds are usually a childhood problem, a scary but minor bout with broken blood vessels just inside the nose. They're caused by a cold, frequent nose blowing and picking, allergies, a dry environment, using too much nasal spray, or a punch or other blow to the nose.

Not all nosebleeds are minor. Some are serious, such as heavy bleeding from deep within the nose (called a posterior nosebleed) that's hard to stop. This type usually strikes the elderly and is most commonly caused by hardening of nasal blood vessels, high blood pressure, medicines to treat blood clots, primary bleeding disorders like hemophilia, or by a tumor in the nose.

Questions To Ask

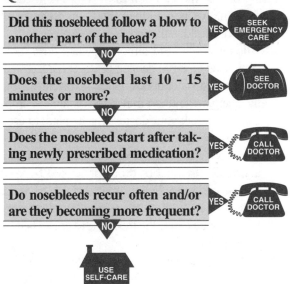

Did this nosebleed follow a blow to another part of the head? YES → SEEK EMERGENCY CARE

NO ↓

Does the nosebleed last 10 - 15 minutes or more? YES → SEE DOCTOR

NO ↓

Does the nosebleed start after taking newly prescribed medication? YES → CALL DOCTOR

NO ↓

Do nosebleeds recur often and/or are they becoming more frequent? YES → CALL DOCTOR

NO ↓

USE SELF-CARE

Self-Care Tips

Although there are lots of ideas about how to treat minor nosebleeds, the following procedure is recommended by the American Academy of Otolaryngology, (Head and Neck Surgery).

- Sit with your head leaning forward.
- Pinch the nostrils shut, using your thumb and forefinger in such a way that the nasal septum (the nose's midsection) is being gently squeezed.

Self-Care Tips continued on next page

Nosebleeds, continued

- Hold for 15 uninterrupted minutes, breathing through your mouth.
- At the same time, apply cold compresses (such as ice in a soft cloth) to the area around the nose.
- For the next 24 hours, make sure your head is elevated above the level of your heart.
- Also, wait 24 hours before blowing your nose, lifting heavy objects, or exercising strenuously.

[Note: If you are unable to stop a nosebleed by using the Self-Care Tips, call your doctor.

Pinkeye

Pinkeye is an inflammation of the conjunctiva, the underside of both the upper and lower eyelids and the covering of the white portion of the eye. The medical term for pinkeye is conjunctivitis. Some causes of pinkeye and solutions that go with them are:

- Allergic reaction to airborne pollen, dust, mold spores, and animal dander, or direct contact with chlorinated water or cosmetics. If you can't avoid the allergens, antihistamines and certain eye drops can help. (Ask your doctor which one(s) to use).
- Bacterial conjunctivitis is characterized by a pus-like discharge. Warm compresses along with an antibiotic ointment or drops prescribed by your doctor can help. When treated right, bacterial conjunctivitis will clear up in two to three days but continue to use the medicine as prescribed by your doctor.
- Viral conjunctivitis is a complication of a cold or flu. This type has less discharge but more tearing than the bacterial form. Antibiotics don't work. Viral conjunctivitis can take 14 to 21 days to clear up.

Questions To Ask

Do you have severe eye pain or are your eyes sensitive to light? YES SEEK EMERGENCY CARE

NO

flowchart continued in next column

Do you have a pus-like discharge that is yellowish-green in color? YES SEE DOCTOR

NO

Have you tried Self-Care Tips and show no improvement after 24 hours or are the symptoms worse? YES CALL DOCTOR

NO

 USE SELF-CARE

Self-Care Tips

Here are some ways to relieve the symptoms of pinkeye:

- Don't touch the eye area with your fingers. If you must wipe your eyes, use tissues.
- With your eyes closed, apply a washcloth soaked in warm (not hot) water to the affected eye three to four times a day for at least 5 minutes at a time. (These soaks also help to dissolve the crusty residue of pinkeye).
- Use over-the-counter eye drops. They may soothe irritation and help relieve itching.
- Avoid wearing eye makeup until the infection has completely cleared up. Never share makeup with others.
- Don't cover or patch the eye. This can make the infection grow.
- Don't wear contact lenses while your eyes are infected.
- Wash your hands often and use your own towels. Pinkeye is very contagious and can be spread from one person to another by contaminated fingers, washcloths, or towels.

Sinus Problems

Your sinuses are behind your cheekbones and forehead, and around your eyes. Healthy sinuses drain almost a quart of mucus every day. They keep the air you breathe wet. Your sinuses can't drain right if they are infected and swollen. Your chances of getting a sinus infection increases if you:

Sinus Problems, continued

- ▭ Have hay fever.
  Smoke.
- ▭ Have a nasal deformity or sinuses that don't drain well.
- ▭ Have an abscess in an upper tooth.
- ▭ Sneeze hard with your mouth closed or blow your nose too much when you have a cold.

Symptoms of a sinus infection are:
- ▭ Head congestion.
- ▭ Nasal congestion and discharge (usually yellowish green).
- ▭ Pain and tenderness over the facial sinuses.
- ▭ Pain in the upper jaw.
- ▭ Recurrent headache that changes with head position and disappears shortly after getting out of bed.
- ▭ Fever.

Sinus complications can be serious. Your doctor can tell if you have a sinus infection with a physical exam, a laboratory study of a sample of your nasal discharge and X-rays of the sinuses. You may need prescriptions for an antibiotic, a decongestant as well as a nasal spray and/or nose drops. These work to clear the infection and reduce congestion. (Severe cases may require surgery to drain the sinuses).

Questions To Ask

Do you have two or more of the following?
- **A fever over 101°F**
- **Greenish-yellow or bloody colored nasal discharge**
- **Severe headache which doesn't get better when you take aspirin or acetaminophen or that is worse in the morning or when bending forward**
- **Pain between the nose and lower eyelid**
- **A feeling of pressure inside the head**
- **Eye pain, blurred vision or changes in vision**
- **Cheek or upper jaw pain**
- **Swelling around the eyes, nose, cheeks and forehead**

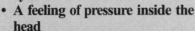 YES → SEE DOCTOR

NO → USE SELF-CARE

Self-Care Tips

A cool-mist humidifier can help. Wet air helps make mucus thin. You can put a warm washcloth or compress on your face, too. This can help with the pain. Here are some more tips:

- ▭ Drink plenty of water and other liquids.
- ▭ Take aspirin or acetaminophen, ibuprofen or naproxen sodium for pain. *[Note: Do not give aspirin or any medication containing salicylates to anyone 19 years of age or younger, unless directed by a physician, due to its association with Reye's Syndrome, a potentially fatal condition.]*
- ▭ Take an over-the-counter decongestant pill, or an over-the-counter pill for pain that also has a decongestant such as Tylenol Sinus. *[Note: Older men should check with their doctor before taking decongestants. Decongestants that have ephedrine can give older men urinary problems.]*

Self-Care Tips continued on next page

Sinus Problems, continued

▭ Use nose drops for only the number of days prescribed. Repeated use of them creates a dependency. Your nasal passages "forget" how to work on their own and you have to continue using drops to keep nasal passages clear. To avoid picking up germs, never borrow nose drops from others. Don't let anyone else use yours, either. Throw the drops away after treatment.

Sore Throats

Sore throats range from a mere scratch to pain so severe that even swallowing saliva hurts. They can be caused by heavy cigarette smoking and infections of the throat, tonsils or nasal passages from a virus, fungus, or bacteria such as the one that causes strep throat.

If an infection is the cause, your doctor may take a throat culture. If streptococcus or any other type of bacteria is the culprit, he or she will prescribe an antibiotic. Be sure you take all of the antibiotic.

If strep throat is left untreated, serious complications, including abscesses, kidney inflammation, or rheumatic heart disease, could arise. An anti-fungal medicine is used to treat a fungal infection.

Questions to Ask

Is it very hard for you to breathe, are you unable to swallow your own saliva, or are you unable to say more than 3 or 4 words between breaths? YES ▸ SEEK EMERGENCY CARE

NO ▾

flowchart continued in next column

Do you have any of the following problems with the sore throat?
- **Fever**
- **Swollen, enlarged neck glands**
- **Headache**
- **General aching feeling**
- **Ear pain**
- **Bad breath**
- **Skin rash**
- **Loss of appetite**
- **Vomiting**
- **Abdominal pain**
- **Chest pain**
- **Dark urine**

YES ▸ SEE DOCTOR

NO ▾

Do the tonsils or back of the throat look bright red or have visible pus deposits? YES ▸ SEE DOCTOR

NO ▾

Does someone else in the family have a strep throat or do you get strep throat often? YES ▸ CALL DOCTOR

NO ▾

Has even a mild sore throat lasted more than 2 weeks? YES ▸ CALL DOCTOR

NO ▾

USE SELF-CARE

Self-Care Tips

How to relieve sore throat discomfort:

▭ Gargle every few hours with a solution of 1/4 teaspoon of salt dissolved in 1/2 cup of warm water.

▭ Drink plenty of warm beverages, such as tea with lemon (with or without honey) and soup.

▭ For strep throat, eat and drink cold foods and liquids such as frozen yogurt, popsicles and ice water.

▭ Use a cool-mist vaporizer or humidifier in the room where you spend most of your time.

▭ Don't smoke.

▭ Avoid eating spicy foods.

Sore Throats, continued

- ☐ Suck on a piece of hard candy or medicated lozenge every so often. (Do not give to children under age 5).
- ☐ Take aspirin or acetaminophen for the pain or fever (or both). *[Note: Do not give aspirin or any medication containing salicylates to anyone 19 years of age or younger unless directed by a physician, due to its association with Reye's Syndrome, a potentially fatal condition.]*
- ☐ Do not get in close contact with anyone you know has a sore throat.

Sty

A sty is a small boil or bacterial infection in a tiny gland of the eyelid.. If the oil-producing glands on the upper or lower rim of the eyelid become infected, they become swollen and painful. A sty is tiny at first, but it can blossom into a bright red, painful sore.

Eventually, a "baby" sty will come to a head and appear yellow, because it accumulates pus. Generally, the tip will face outward, and the sty will break open and drain on its own.

Questions To Ask

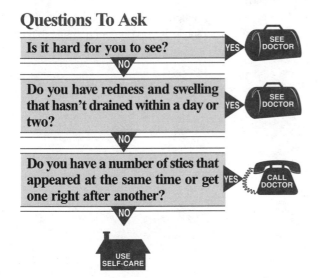

Is it hard for you to see?	YES → SEE DOCTOR
NO ↓	
Do you have redness and swelling that hasn't drained within a day or two?	YES → SEE DOCTOR
NO ↓	
Do you have a number of sties that appeared at the same time or get one right after another?	YES → CALL DOCTOR
NO ↓	
USE SELF-CARE	

Self-Care Tips

You can relieve the discomfort of a sty by following these steps:

- ☐ Apply warm, (not hot), wet compresses to the affected area three or four times a day for 5 to 10 minutes at a time.
- ☐ Avoid situations that expose your eyes to excessive dust or dirt.
- ☐ Don't poke or squeeze the infected area, no matter how tempted you may be to pop the sty. Most sties respond well to home care and don't require further treatment.

Tinnitus (Ringing in the Ears)

Imagine hearing a ringing noise in your ears or head that doesn't go away. This maddening noise, called tinnitus, can range in volume from a ring to a roar. It affects nearly 36 million Americans, most of them older adults. Seven million people are so seriously bothered by tinnitus that living a normal life is not possible. Tinnitus can, in fact, interfere with work, sleep, and normal communication with others.

Like a toothache, tinnitus isn't a disease in itself, but a symptom of another problem. Examples are:

- ☐ Ear wax blocking the ear canals.
- ☐ Food allergies.
- ☐ Reactions to medications.
- ☐ Middle-ear trauma or infections.
- ☐ Blood vessel abnormalities in the brain.
- ☐ Ear nerve damage due to exposure to loud noise.
- ☐ Anemia.
- ☐ Meniere's disease.
- ☐ Diabetes.
- ☐ Brain tumors (rarely).

And sometimes, tinnitus is due simply to advancing age. It often accompanies loss of hearing. Often, tinnitus is temporary and will not lead to deafness. Treatment is aimed at finding and treating the problem that causes the tinnitus.

Tinnitus, continued

Questions to Ask

Do you have severe pain in the ears, forehead or over the cheekbones, a severe headache, dizziness and/or sudden loss of hearing?

NO

Have you been taking aspirin, or other medications containing salicylates such as Trilisate or Disalcid (which are sometimes used to treat arthritis). And do you have these problems with ringing in the ears?
- Nausea
- Vomiting
- Dizziness
- Rapid breathing
- Hallucinations

NO

Along with ringing in the ears, do you have one or more of the following?
- Dizziness
- Vertigo
- Unsteadiness in walking
- Loss of balance
- Vomiting
- Sudden hearing loss

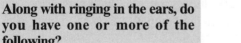

NO

Self-Care Tips

- For mild cases of tinnitus, play the radio or a white noise tape (white noise is a low, constant sound) in the background to help mask the tinnitus.
- Biofeedback or other relaxation techniques can help you calm down and concentrate, shifting your attention away from the tinnitus. Relaxation can reduce stress, which can aggravate tinnitus.
- Exercise regularly to promote good blood circulation.
- Ask your doctor or a Certified Audiologist about a recently developed tinnitus masker, which looks like a hearing aid. Worn on the ear, it makes a subtle noise that masks the tinnitus without interfering with hearing and speech.
- If the noises started during or after traveling in an airplane, try pinching your nostrils and blowing through your nose. Chewing gum or sucking on hard candy may help prevent the popping and ringing sounds in the ear from happening when you do fly. Also, it is prudent to avoid flying when you have an upper respiratory tract or ear infection.
- Limit your intake of caffeine, alcohol, nicotine and aspirin.
- Wear earplugs when exposed to loud noises such as heavy machinery etc., to prevent damage to the ear.

chapter 11

RESPIRATORY PROBLEMS

Asthma

About ten million Americans suffer the wheezing, chest tightness, and breathing difficulty that typifies asthma. Doctors call it an episodic disease because in most asthmatics acute attacks alternate with symptom-free periods. Asthma is a physical problem, not an emotional one (although stress, anxiety, or frustration can cause asthma to worsen), and it can be severe enough to disrupt people's lives. It is a complex disorder which needs to be treated by a doctor who can monitor its condition.

Asthma cuts down the air flow in the lungs. This makes it hard to breathe and can cause wheezing. *[Note: Other things can cause wheezing, too. Something may be stuck in the throat, or there may be an infection. Always tell your doctor about wheezing, especially if your child has it.]* A variety of triggers can set off asthma attacks:

- Having an upper respiratory tract infection or bronchitis.
- Breathing an allergen like pollen, mold, animal dander, or particles of dust or smoke or other irritants.
- Eating certain foods or taking certain medicines.
- Exercising too hard.
- Breathing cold air.
- Experiencing emotional distress.

Asthma attacks range from mild to severe, so treatment varies. Generally, asthma is too complex to treat with over-the-counter preparations. A doctor should keep track of how you are doing.

He or she may prescribe one or more of these for your asthma:

- Bronchodilators, either in oral, inhaled or aerosol form, which open airways to make breathing easier.
- Steroids, either in oral or aerosol form, to counteract an allergic reaction, and when other medicines are not successful for your asthma.

- Cromolyn sodium to be inhaled before an attack that is triggered by allergies or exercise. This won't work once the attack starts. When used with steroids, though, it may help prevent asthma attacks.
- Peak flow meter for home monitoring of asthma.

Questions To Ask

Is it so hard for you to breathe that you can't talk (say 4 or 5 words between breaths) or does your chest feel tight or do you have wheezing that doesn't go away? **YES**

NO

Does your asthma attack not respond to home treatment or prescribed medicine? **YES**

NO

Do you have signs of an infection such as fever, or are you coughing up anything that is green, yellow, or bloody colored? **YES**

NO

Are your asthma attacks coming more often or getting worse? **YES**

NO

Self-Care Tips

Asthmatics can do a number of things to help themselves.

- Drink plenty of liquids (2 to 3 quarts a day) to keep secretions loose.
- Find out what triggers your asthma, and get rid of things that bother you at home and at work.

Self-Care Tips continued on next page

- [ ] Make a special effort to keep your bedroom allergen-free.
  - Sleep with a foam or cotton pillow, not a feather pillow.
  - Use a plastic cover on your mattress.
  - Wash mattress pads in hot water every week.
  - Use throw rugs not carpeting.
  - Don't use drapes.
  - Vacuum and dust often. Wear a dust filter mask when you do.
- [ ] Avoid using perfumes.
- [ ] Don't smoke. Try to stay away from air pollution.
- [ ] Wear a scarf around your mouth and nose when you are outside in cold weather. Doing so will warm the air as you breathe it in and will prevent cold air from reaching sensitive airways.
- [ ] Stop exercising if you start to wheeze.
- [ ] Don't take foods or medicines that have sulfites. Sulfites are in wine and many shellfish. They bother many people with asthma.
- [ ] Sit up during an asthma attack. Don't lie down.
- [ ] Put an electronic air filter in your central heat or air conditioning or use portable air cleaners to keep the air clean.
- [ ] Change and/or wash furnace and air conditioner filters regularly. If you use a portable humidifier or vaporizer, use distilled, not tap water. Clean and dry the appliance after each use.
- [ ] Keep your asthma medicine handy. Take it as soon as you start to feel an attack.
- [ ] Some people with asthma are allergic to aspirin. Use acetaminophen instead.

Bronchitis

If you've ever had a cough that felt as though it started down in your toes, or if you've ever had uncontrollable coughing fits, you may have had bronchitis. Bronchitis can be either acute or chronic, depending on how long it lasts and how serious the damage.

Acute bronchitis is generally caused by an infectious agent (like a virus or bacteria), or an environmental pollutant (like tobacco smoke) that attacks the mucous membranes within the windpipe or air passages in your respiratory tract, leaving them red and inflamed. This type often develops in the wake of a sinus infection, cold, or other respiratory infection, and can last anywhere from three days to three weeks.

Signs of acute bronchitis are:
- [ ] Cough that has little or no sputum.
- [ ] Chills, low-grade fever (usually less than 101°F).
- [ ] Sore throat and muscle aches.
- [ ] Feeling of pressure behind the breastbone or a burning feeling in the chest.

Treatment may include a doctor's prescription for:
- [ ] Bronchodilators (medicines that open up the bronchial passages).
- [ ] Antibiotics.

Chronic bronchitis is usually the result of repeated irritation (or infection) in the bronchial tubes, (the passageways for air moving to and from the lungs). The underlying culprit is most often tobacco smoke. **In fact, cigarette smoking is the most common cause of chronic bronchitis.** So, quitting is essential and may bring complete relief. Other culprits include allergens and air pollution.

Many people, most of them smokers, develop emphysema (destruction of the air sacs) along with chronic bronchitis. Because chronic bronchitis results in abnormal air exchange in the lung and causes permanent damage to the respiratory tract, it's much more serious than acute bronchitis. Chronic bronchitis is not contagious.

Signs of chronic bronchitis are:
- [ ] A cough that brings up mucus or phlegm, for as long as three months or more, for more than two years in a row.

Bronchitis, continued

- ▭ Shortness of breath upon exertion (in early stages).
- ▭ Shortness of breath at rest (in later stages).

Treatment includes:
- ▭ Stopping smoking and avoiding second hand smoke.
- ▭ Avoiding or reducing exposure to air pollution and chemical irritants.
- ▭ Avoiding exposure to cold, wet weather.
- ▭ Using cough medicines with an expectorant.

Questions To Ask

Is the person who has the cough unable to speak more than 4-5 words between breaths or does he or she have purple lips? **YES**

NO

Does the cough occur in a baby and make the baby unable to eat or take a bottle because he or she has a hard time breathing? **YES**

NO

Does the cough occur in an infant less than 3 months old? **YES**

NO

Does it occur in an infant or young child with rapid breathing and sound like a seal's bark? **YES**

NO

Are any of these symptoms also present?
- Fever of 101°F or higher
- Blood in sputum
- Increase in chest pain
- Shortness of breath at rest and at non-coughing times
- Vomiting

YES

NO

flowchart continued in next column

Have you been exposed to chemicals at work or at home, such as those in new carpet or tobacco smoke, etc.? **YES**

NO

Self-Care Tips

- ▭ Breathe air from a cool-mist vaporizer or humidifier. Note though, that vaporizers and humidifiers can harbor bacteria, so they should be cleaned after each use. Inhaling bacteria-laden mist may aggravate bronchitis. Use distilled, not tap water, in the vaporizer.
- ▭ Take aspirin, ibuprofen, acetaminophen or naproxen sodium for fever and aches. *[Note: Do not give aspirin or any medication containing salicylates to anyone 19 years of age or younger unless directed by a physician, due to its association with Reye's Syndrome, a potentially fatal condition.]*
- ▭ Rest.
- ▭ Drink plenty of liquids.
- ▭ Don't smoke.
- ▭ Reduce your exposure to air pollution. (Use air conditioning, air filters, and a mouth and nose filter mask if you have to). If you develop bronchitis easily, stay indoors during episodes of heavy air pollution.
- ▭ Instead of using cough suppressants, use expectorants. Take bronchodilators and antibiotics as prescribed by your doctor.

Common Cold

About 30 million Americans are coughing, sneezing, and blowing their noses while you read this. What's wrong with them? They have the most common illness we know, the common cold. The common cold usually lasts 3 to 7 days and the average person gets 3 or 4 colds a year.

Common Cold, continued

The things that come with a cold are:

- ☐ Sneezing.
- ☐ Runny nose.
- ☐ Fever of 101°F or less.
- ☐ Sore throat.
- ☐ Dry cough.

How do we get colds? Colds are caused by viruses. You can get a cold virus from mucus on a person's hands when they have a cold, such as through a hand shake. You can also pick up the viruses on towels, telephones, money, etc. Then someone else picks them up from you. It goes on and on. Cold viruses also travel through coughs and sneezes.

Prevention

- ☐ Wash your hands often. Keep them away from your nose, eyes, and mouth.
- ☐ Try not to touch people or their things when they have a cold, especially the first 2-3 days they have the cold. This is the most contagious stage.
- ☐ Get lots of exercise. Eat and sleep well.
- ☐ Use a handkerchief or tissues when you sneeze, cough, or blow your nose. This helps keep you from passing cold viruses to others.
- ☐ Use a "cool mist" vaporizer in your bedroom in the winter.

Questions to Ask

Are any of these problems present with the cold?
- **Chest pain that doesn't go away**
- **Quick breathing or trouble breathing**
- **Wheezing**
- **Feeling weak or with no energy**
- **Delirium - delirium can make you restless or confused. Sometimes you see things that aren't there**

YES → SEE DOCTOR

NO

flowchart continued in next column

Do you have any of these problems with the cold?
- **Earache**
- **Bright red sore throat, or sore throat with white spots**
- **Coughing for 10 or more days**
- **Coughing up something that is thick, yellow-green, gray or rust colored**
- **Fever of 104°F in a child under 12 years old**
- **Fever of over 103°F in an adult, under 50 years old**
- **Fever of 102°F or greater in a person 50-60 years old**
- **Fever of 101°F or greater in a person over 60 years old**
- **A bad smell from the throat, nose or ears**

YES → SEE DOCTOR

NO

Do you have pain or swelling over your sinuses that gets worse when you bend over or move your head, especially with a fever of 101°F or higher.

YES → SEE DOCTOR

NO

USE SELF-CARE

Self-Care Tips

Time is the only cure for a cold. These things may make you feel better.

- ☐ Rest in bed if you have a fever.
- ☐ Drink lots of liquids. They help clear out your respiratory tract. This can help prevent other problems, like bronchitis.
- ☐ Take aspirin, acetaminophen, ibuprofen or naproxen sodium for muscle aches and pains. *[Note: Do not give aspirin or any medication containing salicylates to anyone 19 years of age or younger, unless directed by a physician, due to its association with Reye's Syndrome, a potentially fatal condition.]*

Self-Care Tips continued on next page

72

Common Cold, continued

- Use salt water drops to relieve nasal congestion. Mix 1/2 teaspoon of salt in 1 cup of warm water. Place in a clean container. Put 3 to 4 drops into each nostril several times a day, with a clean medicine dropper.

If you have a sore throat:

- Gargle every few hours with a solution of 1/4 teaspoon of salt dissolved in 1/2 cup of warm water.
- Drink tea with lemon (with or without honey).
- Suck on a piece of hard candy or medicated lozenge every so often. (Do not give to children under age 5).
- Use a cool-mist vaporizer or humidifier to add moisture to the air.
- Have chicken soup. It helps clear out mucus.
- Check with your doctor before trying vitamin C. It seems to make some people feel better when they have a cold and may help keep them from getting a cold, even though this has never been medically proven.

Coughs

A lot of things can make you cough:
- An infection.
- An allergy.
- Cigarette smoke.
- Something stuck in your windpipe.
- Dry air.

Coughing can be a sign of many ailments. Your body uses coughing to clear your lungs and airways. Coughing itself is not the problem. What causes the cough is the problem. There are 3 kinds of coughs:
- Productive - A productive cough brings up mucus or phlegm.
- Non-productive - A non-productive cough is dry. It doesn't bring up any mucus.
- Reflex - A reflex cough comes from a problem somewhere else, like the ear or stomach.

How to treat your cough depends on what kind it is, what caused it, and your other symptoms. Treat the cause and soothe the irritation. Stay away from smoking and secondhand smoke, especially when you have a cough. Smoke hurts your lungs and makes it harder for your body to fight infection.

Questions to Ask

Do you have any of these problems?
- **Trouble breathing and not able to say more than 4-5 words between breaths (a baby or small child may be unable to cry, eat or drink a bottle)**
- **Chest pain that travels to the neck, arm, or jaw**
- **Fainting**
- **Coughing up blood**

 YES → SEEK EMERGENCY CARE

NO

Is the person who has the cough a baby or small child? If so, does he or she have these problems, too?
- **The cough sounds like a seal's bark (high and whistling)**
- **A fever of 102°F to 103°F**

 YES → SEE DOCTOR

NO

Did the cough start suddenly and last an hour or more without stopping?

 YES → SEE DOCTOR

NO

Do wheezing, shortness of breath, rapid breathing or swelling of the abdomen, legs and ankles accompany the cough?

 YES → SEE DOCTOR

NO

If the person with the cough is an adult, is there a fever of 102°F or higher?

 YES → SEE DOCTOR

NO

Do you have any of these problems with the cough?
- **Weight loss for no reason**
- **Feeling tired**
- **A lot of sweating at night**

 YES → SEE DOCTOR

NO

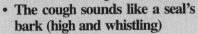

flowchart continued on next page

Coughs, continued

Does your chest hurt only when you cough and does the pain go away when you sit up or lean forward? YES SEE DOCTOR

NO

Do you cough up something thick and green, yellow, or rust-colored, with or without an odor? YES SEE DOCTOR

NO

Has the cough lasted more than 2 weeks without getting better? YES CALL DOCTOR

NO

USE SELF-CARE

Self-Care Tips

For productive coughs (coughs that bring up mucus):

- Drink plenty of liquids. Water helps loosen mucus and soothe a sore throat. Fruit juices are good, too.
- Use a cool-mist vaporizer, especially in the bedroom. Put a humidifier on the furnace.
- Take a shower. The steam can help thin the mucus.
- Ask your pharmacist for an over-the-counter expectorant. Robitussin is one kind.
- Stop smoking cigarettes, cigars, and/or pipes. Stay away from places where people smoke.

For non-productive coughs (coughs that are dry):

- Drink plenty of liquids.
- Drink hot drinks like tea with lemon and honey to soothe the throat.
- Suck on cough drops or hard candy. (Don't give these to children under 5 years of age).
- Take an over-the-counter cough medicine that has dextromethorphan. Robitussin-DM is one of these.
- Try a decongestant if you have post-nasal drip.
- Make your own cough medicine. Mix one part lemon juice and two parts honey. (Don't give this to children less than 1 year old).

Other tips include:

- Don't give children under 5 years of age small objects like paper clips and buttons or foods like peanuts and popcorn. A small child can easily get something caught in their throat or windpipe. Even adults should be careful to chew and swallow foods slowly so they don't "go down the wrong way."
- Don't smoke. Stay away from second-hand smoke.
- Stay away from chemical gases that can hurt your lungs.

Flu

"Oh, it's just a touch of the flu," some say, as if they had nothing more than a cold. Yet each year, 50,000 people die from pneumonia and other complications of the influenza virus, or flu.

Cold and flu symptoms resemble each other, but they differ in intensity. A cold generally starts out with some minor sniffling and sneezing, but the flu hits you all at once. You're fine one hour and in bed the next. A cold rarely moves into the lungs. The flu can cause pneumonia. You may be able to drag yourself to work with a cold, but with the flu you may be too ill to leave your bed.

If the following symptoms come on suddenly and intensely, you probably have the flu:

- Dry cough.
- Sore throat.
- Severe headache.
- General muscle aches or backache.
- Extreme fatigue.
- Chills.
- Fever up to 104°F.
- Pain when you move your eyes, or a burning sensation in the eyes.

Muscle aches and fatigue are the most common signs of the flu. These are normally absent with a cold.

Flu, continued

Prevention

To avoid getting the flu in the first place, medical authorities recommend an influenza vaccination before each flu season for people over age 65 or anyone with a chronic medical illness that would hinder their ability to fight off the flu on their own. The influenza vaccine should be given in September, October or November of each year. Also, get plenty of rest, eat well, and exercise regularly to stay strong and fight off the flu.

The anti-viral medicines amantadine or rimantadine may be prescribed. *[Note: In order for rimantadine to be effective, it must be taken within the first 48 hours of the onset of symptoms of the flu.]* Antibiotics (to combat any bacterial infection, if also present) may also be prescribed by your doctor.

Questions To Ask

Do you have any of these problems with the flu?
- **Inability to speak more than 4 or 5 words between breaths**
- **Purple lips**
- **Chest pain**
- **Spitting up blood**
- **Fever, stiff neck and lethargy**

YES → 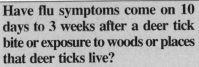 SEEK EMERGENCY CARE

NO ↓

Do you have any of these problems with the flu?
- **Earache**
- **Sinus pain**
- **Something thick coming from the nose, ears, or chest**

YES → 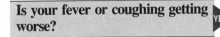 SEE DOCTOR

NO ↓

Is your fever or coughing getting worse?

YES → CALL DOCTOR

NO ↓

Have flu symptoms come on 10 days to 3 weeks after a deer tick bite or exposure to woods or places that deer ticks live?

YES → CALL DOCTOR

NO ↓

flowchart continued in next column

Have you had the flu more than a week and not felt better with any self-care tips? Or have new symptoms developed?

YES → CALL DOCTOR

NO ↓

Have you had any side effects from taking any prescribed or over-the-counter medicines?

YES → CALL DOCTOR

NO ↓

 USE SELF-CARE

Self-Care Tips

There's no cure for the flu. It has to run its course. The goal then, is to minimize discomfort and prevent complications. Generally, if you are in good health, you can treat the flu on your own. The best way to do that is to get plenty of rest, so your body can fight off the virus. Try these tips too:

- Drink lots of hot (not scalding) drinks. They soothe your throat, help unplug your nose and put back water you lose by sweating.

- Gargle with warm, strong tea or warm, salt water. Dissolve 1/4 teaspoon of salt in 1/2 cup of water. Suck on lozenges or hard candies to lubricate your throat. (Don't give these to children under age 5).

- Let yourself cough if you are bringing up mucus.

- Don't suppress a cough that produces mucus. Ask your pharmacist for an over-the-counter expectorant if this is all right with your doctor. Also, if mucus is bloody, yellow or green, contact your physician for advice.

- Don't drink milk or eat dairy products for a couple of days. They make mucus thick and hard to cough up in some persons.

- Wash your hands often, especially after blowing your nose and before handling food. This also helps you avoid spreading the flu virus to others.

- Take a regular dose of acetaminophen, aspirin, ibuprofen or naproxen sodium. *[Note: Do not give aspirin or any medication containing salicylates to anyone 19 years of age or younger unless directed by a physician, due to its association with Reye's Syndrome, a potentially fatal condition.]*

chapter 12
SKIN PROBLEMS

Acne

Acne is a skin condition marked by pimples, such as white heads, blackheads, or even raised, red ones that hurt. These pimples show up on the face, neck, shoulders, and/or back. Acne mostly strikes teenagers and young adults. For some, acne, or the scars it can leave, persist into adulthood. Acne results when oil ducts below the skin get clogged with secretions and bacteria. Factors that help cause acne include:

- Normal increase in the levels of the hormone androgen during adolescence.
- Changes in hormone levels before a woman's menstrual period or during pregnancy.
- Rich moisturizing lotions or heavy or greasy makeup.
- Emotional stress.
- Nutritional supplements that have iodine.
- Cooking oils, tar, or creosote in the air. Creosote is often used as a wood preservative.
- Putting pressure on the face by sleeping on one side of the face or resting your head in your hands.
- Birth control pills, steroids, anti-convulsive medications, and lithium (used to treat some forms of depression).

Most cases of acne can be treated with the self-care tips in the next column. When this is not enough, a doctor can prescribe topical ointments, Retin A cream or gel and/or antibiotics.

Questions To Ask

Is your acne very bad and do you have signs of an infection with it, such as fever and swelling? YES

NO

Are the pimples big and painful? YES

NO

flowchart continued in next column

Have you tried self-care and it doesn't help or does it make your skin worse? YES

NO

USE SELF-CARE

Self-Care Tips

Time is the only real cure for acne, but these tips can help:

- Keep your skin clean. Using a clean washcloth every time, work the soap into your skin gently for a minute or two and rinse well.
- Try an astringent lotion, de-greasing pads, or a face scrub.
- Ask your doctor for the name of a good acne soap.
- Leave your skin alone! Don't squeeze, scratch, or poke at pimples. They can get infected and leave scars.
- Use an over-the-counter lotion or cream that has benzoyl peroxide. (Some people are allergic to benzoyl peroxide. Try a little on your arm first to make sure it doesn't hurt your skin). Follow the directions as listed.
- Wash after you exercise or sweat.
- Wash your hair at least twice a week and keep it off your face.
- For men: Wrap a warm towel around your face before you shave. This will make your beard softer. Always shave the way the hair grows.
- Don't spend too much time in the sun. Don't use a sun lamp.
- Use only water-based makeup. Don't use greasy or oily creams, lotions, or makeups.

Athlete's Foot

It smells bad. It's itchy. It's persistent. It's contagious. And it attacks the skin between the toes (usually the third and fourth). What is it? Fungus of the foot, better known as athlete's foot.

People usually get athlete's foot from walking barefoot over wet floors around swimming pools, locker rooms, and public showers that are contaminated with the fungus, which feasts on moisture. Athlete's foot has these signs and symptoms:

- Moist, soft red or gray-white scales on the feet, especially between the toes.
- Cracked, peeling, dead skin areas.
- Itching.
- Sometimes small blisters on the feet.

Questions To Ask

Do you have signs of athlete's foot and are you diabetic or do you have poor leg circulation? YES

NO ↓

Do you have a fever and/or is the infection spreading or getting worse despite self-treatment described below? YES

NO ↓

Self-Care Tips

If you get athlete's foot:

- Wash your feet twice a day, especially between your toes, and dry the area thoroughly. Do not, however, use deodorant soaps.
- Apply an over-the-counter antifungal powder, cream, or spray between your toes and inside of your socks and shoes.
- Wear clean socks made of cotton or wool. (Natural fibers absorb moisture). Change your socks during the day to help your feet stay dry.

- Wear shoes that provide some ventilation, like sandals or canvas loafers, whenever you can.
- Alternate shoes daily to let each pair air out.

Burns

Burns can result from dry heat (fire), moist heat (steam, hot liquids), electricity, chemicals, or from radiation including sunlight. Treatment for burns depends on:

- The depth of the burn (whether it is first, second, or third degree).
- How much area of the body is affected.
- The location of the burn.

First degree burns affect only the outer skin layer. The skin area appears dry, red, and mildly swollen. A first degree burn is painful and sensitive to touch. Mild sunburn and brief contact with a heat source such as a hot iron are examples of first degree burns. First degree burns should feel better within a day or two. They should heal in about a week if there are no complications. (See self-care tips on page 78).

Second degree burns affect the skin's lower layers as well as the outer skin. They are painful, swollen, and show redness and blisters. The skin also develops a weepy, watery, surface. Examples of second degree burns are severe sunburn, burns caused by hot liquids and a flash from gasoline. Self-care tips can be used to treat many second degree burns depending on their location and how much area is affected. (See "Questions to Ask" and self-care tips on page 78).

Third degree burns affect the outer and deeper skin layers as well as any underlying tissue and organs. They appear black and white and charred. The skin is swollen and underlying tissue is often exposed. The pain felt with third degree burns may be less than with first or second degree burns or none at all because nerve endings may be destroyed. Pain may be felt around the margin of the affected area, however. Third degree burns usually result from electric shocks, burning clothes, severe gasoline fires, etc. They always require emergency treatment. They may result in hospitalization and sometimes require skin grafts.

Burns, continued

Questions to Ask

Is the burn a third degree burn? (Is there absence of pain, charred, black and white skin, and exposure of tissue under the skin? YES	

NO

Is the burn a second degree burn and on the face, hands, feet, genitals or on any joint (elbow, knee, shoulder, etc.)? YES	

NO

Is the burn a second degree burn that has affected more than the outer skin layer, shows signs of blistering, and is extensive (covers more than 3 inches in diameter of the skin)? YES	

NO

Does the burn occur in an infant or a young child? YES	

NO

Self-Care Tips

For First Degree Burns

- Cool the area right away. Place the affected area in a container of cold water or under cold running water. Do this for at least 5 - 10 minutes or until the pain is relieved. This will also reduce the amount of skin damage. (If the affected area is dirty, gently wash it with soapy water first).
- Do not apply ice or cold water for too long a time. This may result in complete numbness lead to frostbite.
- Keep the area uncovered and elevated, if possible. Apply a dry dressing if necessary.
- Do not use butter or other ointments (Example, Vaseline).

- Avoid using local anesthetic sprays and creams. They can slow healing and may lead to allergic reactions in some people.
- Call your doctor if after 2 days you show signs of infection (fever of 101°F or higher, chills, increased redness, swelling, or pus in the infected area) or if the affected area is still painful.
- Take aspirin, acetaminophen, or ibuprofen, or naproxen sodium to relieve pain. *[Note: Do not give aspirin or any medication containing salicylates to anyone 19 years of age or younger, unless directed by a physician, due to its association with Reye's Syndrome, a potentially fatal condition.]*

For Second Degree Burns (that are not extensive and less than 3" in diameter)

- Immerse the affected area in cold (not ice) water until the pain subsides.
- Dip clean cloths in cold water, wring them out and apply them over and over again to the burned area for as long as an hour. Blot the area dry. Do not rub.
- Do not break any blisters that have formed.
- Avoid applying antiseptic sprays, ointments, creams.
- Once dried, dress the area with a single layer of loose gauze that does not stick to the skin. Hold in place with bandage tape that is placed well away from the burned area.
- Change the dressing the next day and every two days after that.
- Prop the burn area higher than the rest of the body, if possible.
- Call your doctor if there are signs of infection (fever of 101°F or higher, chills, increased redness and swelling, and pus) or if the burn shows no sign of improvement after 2 days.

Cold Hands and Feet

Some people wear mittens and heavy socks all year round, even in warm weather, indoors and out. Their hands and feet are always cold. A number of things cause this, such as:

- Poor circulation due to coronary heart disease.
- Raynaud's disease (disorder that affects the flow of blood to the fingers and sometimes to the toes).
- Frostbite.
- Working with vibrating equipment (like a jackhammer)
- A side effect of taking certain medications.
- An underlying disease affecting blood flow in the tiny blood vessels of the skin. (Women smokers may be prone to this last condition).
- Stress.

Symptoms to look for are:

- Fingers or toes turning pale white or blue, then red, in response to cold.
- Tingling or numbness.
- Pain during the white phase of discoloration.

Questions To Ask

Have your hands or feet had prolonged exposure to subfreezing temperatures which may have resulted in frostbite? (Frostbite symptoms are tingling and redness followed by paleness (white or bluish appearance) and numbness of affected areas).

YES → SEEK EMERGENCY CARE

NO ↓

Do your hands or feet turn pale, then blue then red, get painful and numb when exposed to the cold or stress?

YES → CALL DOCTOR

NO ↓

 USE SELF-CARE

Self-Care Tips

If wearing gloves and wool socks and staying indoors where it's warm is a nuisance or doesn't help, try these other warm-up tips:

- Don't smoke. It impairs circulation.
- Avoid caffeine. It constricts blood vessels.
- Avoid handling cold objects. Use ice tongs to pick up ice cubes, for instance.
- With fingers outstretched, swing your arms in large circles, like a baseball pitcher warming up for a game. This may increase blood flow to the fingers. (Skip this tip if you have bursitis or back problems).
- Do not wear footwear that is tight-fitting.
- Wiggle your toes. It may help keep them warm as a result of increased blood flow.
- Practice a relaxation technique, such as biofeedback.

Corns & Calluses

All too often, corns and calluses are the price we pay for neglecting our feet. Corns and calluses are very much alike, they just differ in where they occur.

Corns show up on the bony area on top of the toes and the skin between the toes. Corns feel hard to the touch, are tender, and have a roundish appearance. A small, clear spot called a hen's eye may form in the center.

Calluses can occur on any part of the body that goes through repeated pressure or irritation. Common places are on the balls or heels of the feet, on the hands, and on the knees. Calluses are flat, painless thickenings of the skin.

Corns and calluses form as a protective response. They are extra cells made in a skin area that gets repeated rubbing or squeezing from such things as:

- Footwear that fits poorly.
- Activities that put pressure on the hands, knees and feet.

Corns & Calluses, continued

If self-care tips do not get rid of corns and calluses, a family doctor or foot doctor (podiatrist) may need to be consulted. He or she can scrape away the hardened tissue and peel away the corn with stronger solutions. (Sometimes warts lie underneath corns and need to be treated too).

Questions to Ask

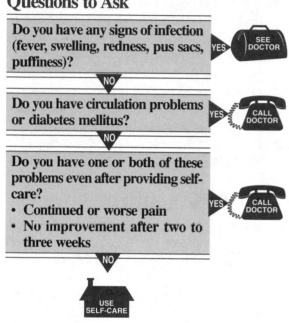

Do you have any signs of infection (fever, swelling, redness, pus sacs, puffiness)? — YES → SEE DOCTOR

NO ↓

Do you have circulation problems or diabetes mellitus? — YES → CALL DOCTOR

NO ↓

Do you have one or both of these problems even after providing self-care?
- Continued or worse pain
- No improvement after two to three weeks

YES → CALL DOCTOR

NO ↓

USE SELF-CARE

Self-Care Tips

For Corns:

Never pick at corns or use toe-nail scissors or clippers, a razor blade or any other sharp tool to cut off corns. You may injure your skin or trigger an infection. Instead:

- Get rid of shoes that fit poorly, especially if they squeeze your toes together.
- Soak your feet in warm water to soften the corn.
- Cover the corn with a protective, non-medicated pad, usually available in drugstores. (A piece of foam rubber or moleskin will do in a pinch).
- If the outer layers of a corn have peeled away, apply a non-prescription liquid of 5 to 10 percent salicylic acid and cover the area with a small bandage.

- Take your shoe to a shoe repair person and ask that he/she sews a metatarsal bar onto your shoe to use when a corn is healing.

For Calluses:

Never try to get rid of a callus by cutting it with a sharp tool. Instead:

- Soak your feet in warm water to soften the callus, and pat dry.
- Rub the callus gently with a pumice stone.
- Cover calluses with protective pads, available in drugstores.
- Check for poorly fitting shoes or other sources of pressure that may lead to calluses.
- Wear gloves if doing a hobby or work that puts pressure on the hands.
- Wear knee pads for activities that puts pressure on your knees.

Cuts, Scrapes & Punctures

Cuts, scrapes, and punctures can all result in bleeding.
- Cuts slice the skin open. Close a cut so it won't get infected.
- Scrapes hurt only the top part of your skin. They can hurt more than cuts, but they heal quicker.
- Punctures stab deep. Leave punctures open so they won't get infected.

You can treat most cuts, scrapes, and punctures yourself. But you should get emergency care if you are bleeding a lot, or if you are hurt very badly. Blood gets thicker after bleeding for a few minutes. This is called clotting. Clotting slows down bleeding. Press on the cut to help slow down the bleeding. You may have to apply pressure for 10 minutes or more for a bad cut. Sometimes a cut needs stitches. Stitches help the cut heal.

Cuts & Scrapes, continued

Questions to Ask

Is the bleeding from the cut, scrape or puncture severe? Has the victim gone into shock? Does blood spurt from the wound? Has a lot of blood been lost? (In an adult, 1/2 cup or more, less in a child). SEEK EMERGENCY CARE

NO

Is there still a lot of bleeding, even though pressure has been applied for 10 minutes or more? SEEK EMERGENCY CARE

NO

Does the cut or puncture have any of these signs?

- The cut or puncture is deep (i.e., appears to go down to the muscle or bone) and/or is located on the scalp or face and require stitches
- The cut is longer than an inch and located on an area of the body that bends, such as the elbow, knee or finger. (Bending will put pressure on the cut)
- The skin on the edges of the cut hangs open
- Bleeding from what seems to be a seemingly minor cut continues after 20 minutes of applied pressure?

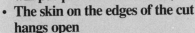 SEEK EMERGENCY CARE

NO

Is the cut or puncture from dirty or contaminated objects, such as rusty nails or objects in the soil, or does the puncture go through a shoe, especially a rubber-soled one? SEEK EMERGENCY CARE

NO

flowchart continued in next column

Did any of these signs of infection appear a day or two after the injury?

- Fever of 101°F or higher
- Redness, swelling, tenderness at and around the site of the wound
- Increased pain
- General ill feeling

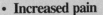 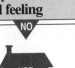 YES SEE DOCTOR

NO

USE SELF-CARE

Self-Care Tips

For cuts and scrapes:

- Clean around the wound with soap and water.
- Press on the cut to stop the bleeding, and continue for up to 10 minutes if you need to. Use a sterile bandage, clean cloth, or if not available, a clean hand. (Try not to use dry gauze. It can stick to the wound). Don't use a band-aid.
- Press on the cut again if it keeps bleeding. Get help if it is still bleeding after 20 or more minutes. Keep pressing on it while you wait for help.
- Lift the part of the body with the cut higher than the person's heart. This slows down blood flow to that spot.
- Apply a first-aid cream, such as Neosporin, or Johnson & Johnson on the cut after it has stopped bleeding and when it is clean and dry. Apply it with a sterile cloth or cotton swab.
- Put one or more band-aids on the cut. Do it this way:
  - Put the band-aid across the cut so it can help hold the cut together.
  - The sides of the cut should touch but not overlap.
  - Don't touch the cut with your hand.
  - You can use a butterfly bandage if you have one.
  - Use more than one bandage for a long cut.
  - For scrapes, make a bandage from gauze and first-aid tape.

Cuts & Scrapes, continued

- Leave the bandage on for 24 hours. Change the bandage every day or two or more often if you need to. Be careful when you take the bandage off. You don't want to make the cut bleed again. If you have used gauze, wet it before you pull it off.
- Take aspirin, acetaminophen, ibuprofen or naproxen sodium for pain. Don't take aspirin every day unless your doctor tells you to, because taking it too much can keep the blood from clotting. *[Note: Do not give aspirin or any medication containing salicylates to anyone 19 years of age or younger, unless directed by a physician, due to its association with Reye's Syndrome, a potentially fatal condition.]*
- Call your doctor or local health department if you have not had a tetanus shot in the last 10 years. (5 years for a deep puncture.)

For punctures that cause minor bleeding:
- Let the wound bleed to clean itself out.
- Remove the object that caused the puncture. Use clean tweezers. Hold a lit match to the ends of the tweezers to sterilize them. *[Note: Don't pull anything out of a puncture wound if blood gushes from it, or if it has been bleeding badly. Get emergency care.]*
- Wash the wound with warm water and soap, or take a bath or shower to clean it.
- Leave the wound open. Cover it with a bandage if it is big or still bleeds a little.
- Soak the wound in warm, soapy water 2 to 3 times a day.

Eczema

Eczema (atopic dermatitis) is a chronic skin condition that usually appears on the scalp, face, neck, or creases of the elbows, wrists, and knees. The symptoms are small blisters and crusty scales on the skin surface, often accompanied by inflammation. Children and adults alike may be affected, and the condition often runs in families. Asthma is often associated with this skin condition.

A variety of irritants or allergens can aggravate eczema, including:
- Wearing wool fabric.
- Sweating.
- Stress.
- Exposure to extreme weather conditions (especially high heat and humidity).
- Eating foods such as eggs, milk, seafood, or wheat products.
- Contact with cosmetics, dyes, medicines, deodorants, skin lotions, permanent press fabrics, and other allergens.

Eczema is quite unpredictable. Usually, it's at its worst in childhood and gradually lets up as you get older. Sometimes it completely disappears for good. Still, eczema can be a lifetime problem.

Questions To Ask

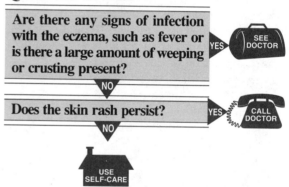

Are there any signs of infection with the eczema, such as fever or is there a large amount of weeping or crusting present? **YES → SEE DOCTOR**

NO ↓

Does the skin rash persist? **YES → CALL DOCTOR**

NO ↓

USE SELF-CARE

Self-Care Tips

True eczema needs a doctor's care. You can, however, do much to maintain good skin care and to manage eczema:
- Bathe less frequently (perhaps sponge bathing in-between tub baths) and add bath oil to the water.
- Or take quick showers.
- Use tepid (not hot) water when bathing or showering.
- Use a mild soap or no soap at all on the areas of eczema.

Eczema, continued

- Avoid contact with wool clothing or blankets.
- After bathing, moisturize your skin with a light, non-greasy, unscented lotion. Avoid lotions that contain alcohol. They can dry the skin.
- Don't overdress or promote perspiration in any way.
- Wear rubber gloves dusted on the inside with talcum powder or cornstarch when doing household chores. Or try cotton-lined latex gloves.
- Avoid any foods, chemicals, cosmetics, or other allergens that worsen the condition.
- And above all, don't scratch! Scratching eczema only makes it worse. You'll break the skin, allowing bacteria to infect the skin. (Keep your fingernails cut short).

Frostbite

Frostbite looks like a serious heat burn, but it's actually body tissue that's frozen and, in severe cases, dead. Most often, frostbite affects the toes, fingers, earlobes, chin, and tip of the nose. These body parts are often left uncovered and can freeze quickly. Danger signs are pain (initially), swelling, white skin, then numbness and eventually loss of function and absence of pain. Blisters may also develop.

Frostbite can happen when temperatures drop below freezing, but wind chill speeds up heat loss and can add to the risk. Frostbite can set in very slowly, or very quickly. This will depend on how long the skin is exposed to the cold and how cold and windy it is.

Prevention

Frostbite can be prevented. Here are some ways to keep warm if you expect to spend any length of time in the cold:

- Layer your clothing. Many layers of thin clothing are warmer than one bulky layer. Air spaces trap body warmth close to the skin, insulating the body against the cold. Wear two or three pairs of socks instead of one heavy pair, for example, and wear roomy shoes.

- Don't drink alcohol or smoke cigarettes. Alcohol causes blood to lose heat quickly. Smoking slows down blood circulation to the extremities.
- Stay indoors as much as possible when it is very cold and windy.
- When you are out of doors, shield your face, etc... from the wind.

Questions To Ask

After being in cold temperature, do you have any of these problems?
- **Swelling of the skin**
- **Loss of function and absence of pain**
- **Skin color changing from white to red to purple**
- **Blisters**
- **Slurred speech**
- **Memory loss**

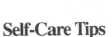

Self-Care Tips

The old wives' tale that says you should treat frostbite by rubbing the area with snow or soaking it in cold water is wrong. This treatment is ineffective and dangerous. Instead:

- Warm the affected area by soaking in a tub of warm water (101°F to 104°F) and an antiseptic solution.
- Stop when the affected area becomes red, not when sensation returns. (This should take about 45 minutes. If done too rapidly, thawing can be painful and blisters may develop.)
- Keep exposed area elevated.
- Never massage a frostbitten area.
- Protect exposed area from the cold. It is more sensitive to re-injury.

Hives

Hives, or urticaria, are red, raised, itchy welts. They appear, sometimes in clusters, on the face, trunk of the body, and, less often, on the scalp, hands, or feet. Like the Cheshire cat in Alice's Adventures in Wonderland, hives can change shape, fade, then rapidly reappear. A single hive lasts less than 24 hours, but after an attack new ones may crop up for up to six weeks. According to estimates, nearly 20 percent of Americans will get hives at some time in their lives.

Hives can be (but aren't always) an allergic response to something you touched, inhaled, or swallowed. Some common causes of hives include:

- Reactions to medications such as aspirin, sulfa, and penicillin.
- Animal dander (especially from cats).
- Cold temperatures.
- Emotional or physical stress (including exercise).
- Foods (especially chocolate, nuts, shellfish, or tomatoes).
- Infections.
- Inhalants (especially pollen, mold spores, or airborne chemicals).
- Insect bites.
- Rubbing or putting pressure on the skin.
- Exposure to chemicals.
- Malignant or connective tissue disease.

Sometimes, it is not known what causes hives. But if you can identify the triggers (try keeping a diary), you may be able to prevent future outbreaks.

Questions To Ask

Do you have any of these problems?
- **Shortness of breath and breathing difficulties**
- **Wheezing, dizziness**
- **Swollen lips, tongue, and/or throat**

 YES SEEK EMERGENCY CARE

NO

flowchart continued in next column

 Did hives start after recently taking a medication? YES CALL DOCTOR

NO

 Do you have itching that is constant, and/or severe or do you have a fever? YES CALL DOCTOR

NO

 USE SELF-CARE

Self-Care Tips

Here are some tips for a case of ordinary, non-threatening hives:

- Don't take hot baths or showers. Heat worsens most rashes and makes them itch more.
- Apply cold compresses or take a warm bath.
- Wear loose-fitting clothing.
- Relax as much as possible. Studies have shown that relaxation therapy and even hypnosis help ease the itching and discomfort of hives.
- Ask your doctor whether or not you should take an antihistamine and have him or her recommend one. Antihistamines can help relieve itching and suppress hives. (Keep in mind that antihistamines can cause drowsiness and may make it dangerous for you to drive or perform other tasks requiring alertness).
- Avoid taking aspirin, ibuprofen or naproxen sodium. These may aggravate hives.

Insect Stings

Warm weather months often include run-ins with bees, wasps, mosquitos, fleas, spiders, etc.

As you'd expect, most people who have been stung know it. The most common symptoms are limited areas of pain and swelling, with redness and itching. Beyond that, the symptoms of bee and wasp stings vary, depending on where you're stung and how sensitive you are to the sting.

Insect Stings, continued

People who are allergic to insect stings may have a severe reaction known as anaphylaxis (even if they've never had an allergic reaction to a sting before). The symptoms of a severe anaphylactic reaction include generalized swelling, wheezing, difficult breathing, a severe drop in blood pressure, and sometimes coma and death. Needless to day, this is a medical emergency, so if you start to have a serious reaction to a sting, get medical help immediately.

If you've ever experienced an allergic reaction to an insect sting in the past, you should carry an emergency medical kit containing epinephrine (a medicine to stop the body-wide reaction) and a hypodermic needle to inject it, an antihistamine, and an identification bracelet that lets others know that you're allergic to insect stings. Also, people who have had severe reactions to bee or wasp stings should consider allergy shots as a protective measure.

Prevention

How can you avoid getting stung?
- Keep foods and drinks tightly covered. (Bees love sweet foods and soft drinks).
- Avoid sweet-smelling colognes. Wear an insect repellent instead.
- Avoid looking like a flower. Choose white or neutral colors that won't attract bees.
- Wear snug clothing that covers your arms and legs, and don't go barefoot.
- Be careful when making home improvements such as removing shutters from the house. Bees often build hives behind shutters.
- Treat animals for fleas.

Questions To Ask

If you are stung by an insect, do you have these problems?
- **Generalized swelling**
- **Throat feels closed up**
- **Wheezing**
- **Difficulty in breathing and/or swallowing**
- **Slurred speech**
- **Confusion**
- **Hives all over the body**

YES

Use "Bee Sting Kit" if you have one

NO

Were you stung in the mouth or on the tongue? YES

NO

Has the bitten area become red, swollen, warm and tender? YES

NO

Have symptoms of soreness, redness, and/or itching not been relieved by self-care tips below? YES

NO

Self-Care Tips

- Gently scrape out the stinger, if there is one, as soon as possible.
- Don't pull or squeeze the stinger. It contains venom, and you'll end up re-stinging yourself. (This applies to bees only; yellow jackets, wasps, and hornets don't lose their stingers).
- Clean the sting area with soapy water.
- Put a cold compress on the sting. Put ice in a cloth, plastic bag or plastic wrap. Don't put ice directly on the skin. Hold the cold compress onto the site for 15-20 minutes.
- Apply ammonia diluted with water to the sting area.

Insect Stings, continued

Take aspirin or acetaminophen, ibuprofen or naproxen sodium for the pain, and/or an antihistamine for the itching and swelling (provided you don't have to avoid these medicines for medical reasons). *[Note: Do not give aspirin or any medication containing salicylates to anyone 19 years of age or younger, unless directed by a physician, due to its association with Reye's Syndrome, a potentially fatal condition.]*

Poison Ivy

During a walk through the woods you can see birds, small animals, and beautiful plants. But if you come in contact with poison ivy along the way, you may leave with an itchy rash as a souvenir of your nature trek.

The rash is caused by urushiol, a resin given off by poison ivy, poison oak, and other related plants. Urushiol is an allergen, not a poison. Not everyone reacts to it. If you're allergic to the resin, however, and either touch the plant directly or come in contact with clothing or pets that have been exposed to it, you'll develop a rash of itchy, oozing blisters, sometimes with swelling.

Prevention

Knowing what poison ivy looks like is the key to prevent getting a rash. The old adage, "Leaflets three, let it be" holds true.

Questions To Ask

Does the rash show signs of infection? Is the skin very bright red or is there pus? **YES** SEE DOCTOR

↓ NO

Has the rash spread to the mouth, eyes, or genitals, or have you had severe reactions to poison ivy (or poison oak) in the past? **YES** SEE DOCTOR

↓ NO

flowchart continued in next column

Are self-care tips not helpful, or is the itching so severe that you can't tolerate it? **YES** CALL DOCTOR

↓ NO

USE SELF-CARE

Self-Care Tips

If you have poison ivy, here's what to do:

- Remove and wash all clothes and shoes that have been contaminated. If an article isn't washable, isolate it in a ventilated area for three weeks.
- Bathe with soap and water, then apply rubbing alcohol to the exposed skin with cotton balls. Rinse with water afterward. Doing this within six hours of being exposed to the poison ivy may prevent a reaction.
- A rash may still develop two or three days after contact with the resin. If that happens, apply calamine lotion or 1% hydrocortisone cream (available over-the-counter).
- Take an oral antihistamine, such as diphenhydramine (brand name Benadryl), to relieve itching.
- If weeping blisters develop, cover them with gauze and keep them wet, with a solution of one tablespoon baking soda in one quart of water. (The fluid in blisters will not cause the rash to spread).

Shingles

Shingles (herpes zoster) is a skin disorder triggered by the chicken pox virus (Varicella zoster) that you first encountered as a child.

This virus is thought to lie dormant in the spinal cord until later in life. Shingles most often occurs between the ages of 50 and 70 in both men and women. Even though shingles is not as contagious as chicken pox, infants and people whose immunity is low, should not be exposed to it. Besides aging, the risks for getting shingles increases with:

Shingles, continued

- Hodgkin's disease or other cancer.
- Any illness in which infection-fighting systems are below par.
- The use of anti-cancer medications or any medications that suppress the immune system (Example: Corticosteroids).
- Stress or trauma, either emotional or physical.

Symptoms of shingles include:
- Pain, itching, or tingling sensation before the rash appears.
- A rash of painful red blisters, which later crust over. Most often, the rash appears on the torso or side of the face. Only one side of the face or body is affected. Shingles is almost never present on both sides of the body. It is serious if it affects the eye, because it can lead to blindness.
- Though rare, fever and general weakness sometimes occur.

After the crusts fall off (usually within three weeks), pain can persist in the area of the rash. This usually goes away on its own after one to six months. Chronic pain can, however, last for months or years. The older you are, the greater the chances are that this is the case and the recovery time may also take longer.

Most cases of shingles are mild but can result in chronic, severe pain, blindness or deafness. So, to be on the safe side, if you get shingles it is wise to let your doctor know.

Treatment for shingles includes:
- Pain relief with analgesics. Codeine may sometimes be prescribed.
- Prescription medicines: Famvir, and acyclovir (Zovirax) oral and/or topical ointment, can be very effective. The sooner these medicines are used, the better the results.
- An antibiotic if the blisters become infected.
- Antihistamines.
- Corticosteroids.
- Tranquilizers for a short time.

Questions to Ask

With shingles, are you over 60 years of age, taking anti-cancer or other immunosuppressive medicines, or have a chronic illness? — YES → SEE DOCTOR

NO ↓

Has the shingles affected your eyes? — YES → SEE DOCTOR

NO ↓

Do the blisters itch uncontrollably or are they very painful? — YES → SEE DOCTOR

NO ↓

Do you have a fever and/or general weakness? — YES → SEE DOCTOR

NO ↓

Do any symptoms of shingles make you uncomfortable? — YES → SEE DOCTOR

NO ↓

USE SELF-CARE

Self-Care Tips

Following are things you can do (along with your doctor's treatment plan) to help relieve an active outbreak of shingles:

- Take an over-the-counter pain reliever such as acetaminophen, aspirin, ibuprofen or naproxen sodium, unless your doctor has given you prescription pain medicine. *[Note: Ask your doctor which over-the-counter pain medicine is best for you.]*
- If possible, keep sores open to the air. Don't bandage them unless you live with or are around children or adults who have not yet had the chicken pox. They could pick up chicken pox from exposure to shingles.
- Don't wear restrictive clothing that irritates the area of the body where sores are present.
- Wash blisters, but never scrub them.
- Apply calamine lotion or baking soda to help alleviate the symptoms.

Self-Care Tips continued on next page

Shingles, continued

- ☐ Avoid drafty areas where you can get chilled.
- ☐ Put cool compresses on the blisters. You can use several things: A cold cloth or towel dipped in ice water, a bag of frozen vegetables or an ice pack wrapped in a thin towel. Put the cool compress on the blisters for 20 minutes at a time.

Skin Rashes

Skin rashes come in all forms and sizes. Some are raised bumps, others are flat red blotches. Some are itchy blisters, and others are patches of rough skin. Most rashes are harmless and clear up on their own within a few days. A few may need medical attention. The skin is one of the first areas of the body to react when exposed to something you or your child is allergic to.

The chart on page 90 lists information on some common skin rashes.

Questions to Ask

| Are you having trouble breathing or swallowing, or is the tongue swollen? | YES | SEEK EMERGENCY CARE |

↓ NO

| Do you have any of the following?
• **Fever**
• **Headache**
• **Sore throat**
• **A fine red rash that feels rough like sandpaper**
• **Joint pain along with a target-like rash** | YES | SEE DOCTOR |

↓ NO

| Are there any large, fluid-filled blisters present or pus or swelling around the rash lesions? | YES | SEE DOCTOR |

↓ NO

| Have you recently been exposed to someone with a "strep" infection? | YES | SEE DOCTOR |

↓ NO

flowchart continued in next column

| If your child has a diaper rash, are there also blisters or small red patches that appear outside the diaper area, such as on the chest? | YES | SEE DOCTOR |

↓ NO

| When the rash started, were you taking any medications or were you stung by an insect? | YES | CALL DOCTOR |

↓ NO

| Is the rash getting worse, keeping you from sleeping and/or do self-care tips not relieve symptoms? | YES | CALL DOCTOR |

↓ NO

USE SELF-CARE

Self-Care Tips

Heat rash is best treated by staying in a cool, dry area. It will usually disappear within 2 to 3 days if you keep the skin cool. Things you can do:

- ☐ Take a bath in cool water, without soap, every couple of hours.
- ☐ Let your skin air dry.
- ☐ Apply calamine (not Caladryl) lotion to the very itchy spots.
- ☐ Put corn starch in body creases (inside elbows, etc.).
- ☐ Don't use ointments and creams that can block the sweat gland pores.

To treat diaper rash in a child:

- ☐ Change diapers as soon as they become wet or soiled (even at night if the rash is extensive).
- ☐ Wash your baby with plenty of warm water, not disposable wipes, to prevent irritating the skin. If the skin appears irritated, apply a light coat of zinc oxide ointment after the skin is completely dry.
- ☐ Keep the skin dry and exposed to air.
- ☐ Before putting on a fresh diaper, keep your baby's bottom naked on a soft, fluffy towel for 10 to 15 minutes.

Skin Rashes, continued

- [ ] Put diapers on loosely so air can circulate under them. If disposable diapers are used, punch a few holes in them. Avoid ones with tight leg bands.
- [ ] Don't use plastic pants until the rash is gone.
- [ ] Wash cloth diapers in mild soap. Add 1/2 cup of vinegar to your rinse water to help remove what's left of the soap.

For temporary relief from the itchy rash typical of poison ivy, oak and sumac:

- [ ] As soon as possible, remove your clothes and shoes. Wash with soap and water to remove the plant oil from the skin. Rub the affected skin area with alcohol or alcohol wipes and then rinse with water. Wash all clothes and shoes you have on.
- [ ] Trim your nails. Try not to scratch. Keep busy with other activities.
- [ ] Soak the rash area in cool water or take baths with Aveeno (an over-the-counter colloidal oatmeal product) or put one cup of oatmeal in a tub full of water.
- [ ] Take a hot shower if tolerated. At first, the itching will get worse, but after a while it stops and the relief can last for hours. Repeat as soon as the itching starts again. Use calamine lotion every three to four hours.
- [ ] Apply a hydrocortisone cream. Put a very small dab of cream on the rash. Be careful not to rub and spread the poison. If you can see the cream on the skin, you've used too much. Repeat as needed every two to four hours. Do not use these creams near the eyes.
- [ ] Learn how to recognize poison ivy, oak and sumac. Stay away from them.

Hives can be eased if you:

- [ ] Take an antihistamine such as Benadryl. Check the labels of cold medications that contain an antihistamine. Those that have diphenhydramine or chlorpheniramine are good choices. Know, though, that most antihistamines are likely to cause drowsiness.
- [ ] Cool off. Rub an ice cube over the hives, drape a washcloth dipped in cool water over the affected areas or take a cool-water bath.
- [ ] Rub your body with Calamine lotion, witch hazel or zinc oxide.
- [ ] Find and eliminate the cause of the allergic reaction.

For cradle cap in babies:

- [ ] Use an anti-dandruff shampoo once a day, massaging your baby's scalp with a soft brush or washcloth for 5 minutes.
- [ ] Soften the hard crusts by applying mineral oil on the scalp before washing your child's hair. Be sure to thoroughly wash the oil out completely. Otherwise, the cradle cap condition may worsen.

To protect yourself from Lyme disease:

- [ ] Wear long pants tucked into socks and long-sleeve shirts when you walk through fields and forests such as when camping. Light colored, tightly woven clothing is best.
- [ ] Inspect yourself for ticks after these outdoor activities.
- [ ] Remove any ticks found on the skin as follows:
  - Use tweezers to grasp the tick as close to the skin as possible.
  - Pull in a steady upward motion.
  - Try not to crush the tick because the secretions released may spread disease.
  - Wash the wound area and your hands with soap and water after removing ticks.
  - Save any removed ticks in a jar and take them to the doctor to aid in the diagnosis of Lyme disease.

COMMON SKIN RASHES

CONDITION OR ILLNESS	CAUSES	WHAT RASH LOOKS LIKE	SKIN AREA(s) AFFECTED	OTHER SYMPTOMS
Diaper Rash	Dampness and the interaction of urine and the skin	Small patches or rough skin, tiny pimples	Buttocks, thighs, genitals	Soreness, no itching
Cradle Cap	Hormones that pass through the placenta before birth	Scaly, crusty rash (in newborns)	Starts behind the ears and spreads to the scalp	Fine, oily scales
Heat Rash (Prickly Heat)	Blocked off sweat glands	Small red pimples, pink blotchy skin	Chest, waist, back, armpits, groin	Itching (may be a result of fever)
[1]Roseola	Herpes virus type-6	Flat, rosy red rash	Chest and abdomen	High fever 2-4 days before rash - child feels only mildly ill during fever
[1]Fifth Disease	Human parvovirus B19	Red rash of varying shades that fades to a flat, lacy pattern (rash comes and goes)	Red rash on facial cheeks, lacy-like rash can also appear on arms and legs	Mild disease with no other symptoms or a slight runny nose and sore throat
Eczema	Allergens	Dry, red, cracked skin, blisters that ooze and crust over, sufficient scratching leads to a thickened rough skin	On cheeks in infants, on neck, wrists, inside elbows, and backs of knees in older children	Moderate to intense itching (may only itch first, then rash appears hours to days later)
[1]Chicken Pox[2]	Varicella/herpes zoster virus	Flat red spots that become raised resembling small pimples. These develop into small blisters that break and crust over	Back, chest and abdomen first, then rest of body	Fatigue and mild fever 24 hours before rash appears - intense itching
[1]Scarlet Fever	Bacterial infection (streptococcal)	Rough, bright red rash (feels like sandpaper)	Face, neck, elbows, armpits, groin (spreads rapidly to entire body)	High fever, weakness before rash, sore throat, peeling of the skin afterward (especially palms)
[1]Impetigo	Bacterial infection of the skin	In infants, pus-filled blisters, and red skin. In older children, golden crusts on red sores	Arms, legs, face and around the nose first, then most of body	Sometimes fever - occasional itching
Hives	Allergic reaction to food, insect bites, viral infection, medicine or other substance	Raised red bumps with pale centers (resemble mosquito bites), shape, size and location of spots can change rapidly	Any area	Itching - in extreme cases, swelling of throat, difficulty breathing (may need emergency care)
Poison Ivy, Oak, Sumac	Interaction of oily resins of plant leaves with skin	Red, swollen skin rash and lines of tiny blisters	Exposed areas	Intense itching and burning
Lyme Disease	Bacterial infection spread by deer tick bite(s)	Red rash that looks like a bull's-eye: raised edges surround the tick bites with pale centers in the middle. Rash starts to fade after a couple of days	Exposed skin areas where ticks bite, often include scalp, neck, armpit and groin	No pain, no itching at time of bite. Fever-rash occurs in the week following the bite(s)

[1] These conditions are contagious

[2] See pages 91 and 129 of this booklet for more information on Chicken Pox

Skin Rashes, continued

The goals in treating chicken pox are to reduce and relieve the itching for comfort and to prevent scratching off the scabs which could start a secondary infection and/or leave scars.

For chicken pox in children:
- Encourage your child not to scratch the scabs.
- Keep him or her busy with other activities.
- Give your child a cool bath without soap, every 3 to 4 hours for the first couple of days at 15 to 20 minutes at a time. Add one-half cup of baking soda or colloidal oatmeal bath packet, such as Aveeno, to the bath water. Pat, do not rub, your child dry. Or, dip a washcloth in cool water and place it on the itchy areas.
- Apply calamine (not caladryl) lotion for temporary relief.
- Trim your child's fingernails to prevent infection caused by opened blisters. Scratching off the crusty scabs may leave permanent scars.
- Cover the hands of infants with cotton socks if they are scratching their sores.
- Wash your child's hands three times a day with an antibacterial soap such as Safeguard or Dial to avoid infecting the open blisters.
- Keep your child cool and calm. Heat and sweating make the itching worse. Also, keep your child out of the sun. Extra chicken pox will occur on parts of the skin exposed to the sun.
- Give your child Benadryl, an over-the-counter antihistamine, if the itching is severe or stops your child from sleeping. (See label for proper dosage).
- Give your child acetaminophen (children's versions of the following: Tylenol, Tempra, Liquiprin, Datril, Anacin 3 or Panadol) for the fever. *[Note: Do not give aspirin or any medication containing salicylates to anyone 19 years of age or younger, unless directed by a physician, due to its association with Reye's Syndrome, a potentially fatal condition.]*
- Give your child soft foods and cold fluids if he or she has sores in the mouth. Do not offer salty foods or citrus fruits that may irritate the sores.
- Have your child gargle with salt water (one-half teaspoon to 8 ounces of water) to help ease itching in the mouth, if necessary.

- Reassure your child that the "bumps" are not serious and will go away in a week or so.

For adults with chicken pox:
- Follow any measures listed above that will bring relief. *[Note: Adults may take longer to recover from chicken pox and are more likely to develop complications. See your doctor if this is the case.]*

For eczema, see self-care tips on page 82.

Sunburn

You should never get sunburned! It is not healthy. It leads to premature aging, wrinkling of the skin and skin cancer.

Sunburn is caused by overexposure to ultraviolet (UV) light. This can be from the sun, sun lamps, or even from some workplace light sources such as welding arcs. Sunburn results in red, swollen, painful, and sometimes blistered skin. Chills, fever, nausea, and vomiting can occur if the sunburn is extensive and severe.

The risk for sunburn is increased for:
- Persons with fair skin, blue eyes, and red or blond hair.
- Persons taking some medications including sulfa medications, tetracyclines, some diuretics and even Benadryl (an over-the-counter antihistamine).
- Persons exposed to industrial UV light sources.
- Persons exposed to excessive outdoor sunlight.

Sunburn can be prevented by using the following measures:
- Avoid the sun's rays during the hours of 10:00 a.m. and 4:00 p.m.
- Use sunscreen with a sun protective factor (SPF) of 15 or more when exposed to the sun. The lighter your skin the higher the SPF number should be. To be effective, sunscreen should be reapplied every hour and after swimming. Make-up for women is now available with sun screen protection.
- Wear a hat when in the sun.

Sunburn, continued

- Wear muted colors such as tan. Brilliant colors and white reflect the sun onto the face. Clothing is now available with sunscreen protection.

Questions to Ask

Are there any of these signs of dehydration?
- **Confusion**
- **Very little or no urine output**
- **Sunken eyes**
- **Skin that is wrinkled or sags**
- **Extreme dryness in the mouth**

YES → SEEK EMERGENCY CARE

NO ↓

Do you have a fever of 102°F or higher or have severe pain or blistering with the sunburn? YES → SEE DOCTOR

NO ↓

USE SELF-CARE

Self-Care Tips

- Cool the affected area with clean towels, cloths or gauze dipped in cool water or take a cool bath or shower.
- Take aspirin, acetaminophen, ibuprofen, or naproxen sodium to relieve pain, headache, and to reduce fever. *[Note: Do not give aspirin or any medication containing salicylates to anyone 19 years of age or younger, unless directed by a physician, due to its association with Reye's Syndrome, a potentially fatal condition.]*
- Use an over-the-counter topical steroid cream such as Cortaid if the pain persists.
- Rest in a comfortable position, in a cool, quiet room.
- Drink plenty of water to replace fluid loss.
- Avoid using local anesthetic creams or sprays (such as benzocaine or Lidocaine) or use sparingly because they cause allergic reactions in some persons.

Varicose Veins

Varicose veins are swollen and twisted veins that look blue and are close to the surface of the skin. They are unsightly and uncomfortable. Veins bulge, throb, and feel heavy. The legs and feet can swell. The skin can itch. Varicose veins may occur in almost any part of the body. They are most often seen in the back of the calf or on the inside of the leg between the groin and the ankle. Hemorrhoids (veins around the anus) can also become varicose. Causes and risk factors for varicose veins include:

- Obesity.
- Pregnancy.
- Hormonal changes at menopause.
- Activities or hobbies that require standing for a long time.
- A family history of varicose veins.
- Past vein diseases such as thrombophlebitis (inflammation of a vein before a blood clot forms).

Medical treatment is not required for most varicose veins unless problems result, such as a deep-vein blood clot or severe bleeding which can be caused by injury to the vein.

Your doctor can take an X-ray of the vein (venogram) and/or a special ultrasound to tell if there are any problems. Surgery can be done to remove enlarged veins. Sclerotherapy can also be done on smaller veins. This procedure uses a chemical injection into the vein that causes it to close up. Other veins then take over its work. Both of these treatments, however, may bring only temporary success, and more varicose veins can develop.

Questions to Ask

Has the varicose vein become swollen, red, very tender or warm to the touch? YES → SEE DOCTOR

NO ↓

flowchart continued on next page

Varicose Veins, continued

Are varicose veins accompanied by a rash or sores on the leg or near the ankle or have they caused circulation problems in your feet?

 YES → SEE DOCTOR

NO ↓

 USE SELF-CARE

Self-Care Tips

To relieve and prevent varicose veins:

- Don't cross your legs when sitting.
- Exercise regularly. Walking is a good choice. It improves leg and vein strength.
- Keep your weight down.
- Avoid standing for prolonged periods of time. If your job or hobby requires you to stand, shift your weight from one leg to the other every few minutes.
- Wear elastic support socks that go up to the knee but do not cover the knee. The top of these socks must not be tight.
- Don't wear clothing or undergarments that are tight or constrict your waist, groin or legs.
- Eat high-fiber foods like bran cereals, whole grain breads, and fresh fruits and vegetables to promote regularity. Drink at least 8 glasses of water a day. These things help prevent constipation. (Constipation contributes to varicose veins).
- To prevent swelling, limit your salt intake.
- Exercise your legs. (From a sitting position, rotate your feet at the ankles, turning them first clockwise, then counterclockwise, using a circular motion. Next, extend your legs forward and point your toes to the ceiling, then to the floor. Then, lift your feet off the floor and gently bend your legs back and forth at the knees).
- Elevate your legs when resting.
- Get up and move about every 35 to 45 minutes when traveling by air or even when sitting in an all day conference. (Opt for an aisle seat in such situations).
- Stop and take short walks at least every 45 minutes when taking long car rides.

chapter 13

DIGESTIVE PROBLEMS

Constipation

Constipation is when you have trouble having bowel movements. Abdominal swelling, straining during bowel movements, hard stools and the feeling of continued fullness even after a bowel movement are also signs of constipation. It can be very uncomfortable, but it usually doesn't signal disease or a serious problem. What things cause or lead to constipation? A number of things do. These include:

- ▢ Not drinking enough fluids.
- ▢ Not eating enough dietary fiber.
- ▢ Not being active enough.
- ▢ Using laxatives over a long period of time.
- ▢ Taking certain medicines (Examples: some heart, pain and anti-depressant medicines as well as antacids, antihistamines, water pills and narcotics).
- ▢ Not going to the bathroom when you have the urge to have a bowel movement.
- ▢ Medical problems such as hemorrhoids or an underactive thyroid gland.

It is important to know that it is not necessary to have a bowel movement daily. What is more important is what is normal for you.

The "cure" for constipation generally consists of correcting the things that make bowel habits irregular. (See Self-Care Tips in the next column). You may also need to discuss measures with your doctor about medications and health conditions that could be causing you to be constipated.

Questions To Ask

Is the constipation accompanied by any of the following?
- **Fever**
- **Severe abdominal pain, especially located in the lower left section**
- **Persistent vomiting**
- **Abdominal bloating**
- **Weight loss**
- **Very thin pencil-like stools or blood seen in the stools**

YES → SEE DOCTOR

NO ↓

Did the constipation occur after taking prescribed or over-the-counter medicines and/or vitamins?

YES → CALL DOCTOR

NO ↓

Do you have persistent constipation despite using the self-care tips listed below?

YES → CALL DOCTOR

NO ↓

 USE SELF-CARE

Self-Care Tips

- ▢ Eat foods high in dietary fiber, like bran, whole-grain breads and cereals and fresh fruits and vegetables daily. They serve as natural stool softeners thanks in part to their fiber content. One type of fiber from these foods absorbs water like a sponge, turning hard stools into large, soft, easy-to-pass masses.
- ▢ Drink at least 1-1/2 to 2 quarts of water and other liquids every day.
- ▢ Drink hot water, tea or coffee. These may help stimulate the bowel.
- ▢ Get plenty of exercise, to help your bowels move things along.

Constipation, continued

- Don't resist the urge to eliminate or put off a trip to the bathroom.
- Keep in mind that medicines such as antacids and iron supplements can be binding. Stay away from them if you get constipated easily. Discuss this with your doctor first.
- If necessary, for occasional constipation, you may need an over-the-counter stool softener, mild laxative or enema. Check with your doctor ahead of time so you'll know what is best for you to take if and when you do get constipated.

Ask your doctor about the use of "bulk-forming" laxatives such as Metamucil, Perdiem or Fiber Con. You may be able to use these daily, if necessary. Start out slowly and gradually increase how much you take. Also drink plenty of liquids with them. Bloating, cramping or gas may be noticed at first, but these symptoms should go away in a few weeks or less.

Do not use "stimulant" laxatives such as Ex-Lax, Dulcolax, Senokot or enemas without your doctor's permission. Short-term use of them may be O.K., but in the long run, they can make you even more constipated, because your intestines can become lazy and may not work as well on their own. Long term use of these laxatives can also lead to a mineral imbalance, make it harder for your body to benefit from medicines, and lower the amount of nutrients you absorb.

Diarrhea

Diarrhea is the frequent passage of watery, loose bowel movements. Almost everyone gets diarrhea once in a while. Usually, it only lasts a day or two, and isn't serious.

Many things can cause diarrhea:
- Infection by viruses, bacteria or parasites.
- Drinking bad water or eating spoiled food.
- Food poisoning.
- Allergies.
- Emotional upset.
- Overuse of laxatives.

- Certain medications, including some antibiotics (like tetracycline, clindamycin, and ampicillin).
- Diverticulitis - a disease in the intestines.
- Inflammatory bowel disease (primarily ulcerative colitis and Crohn's disease).

Questions To Ask

Does the diarrhea occur in an infant or child and is it accompanied by any of the following?
- **Sunken eyes**
- **Dry skin**
- **Dry mouth**
- **Dry diaper for more than 3 hours in an infant**
- **Passing no urine for more than 6 hours in a child**
- **Unusual lethargy, weak cry**
- **Irritability, very upset or cranky**

YES SEEK EMERGENCY CARE

NO ↓

Does an adult have any of these problems with the diarrhea?
- **Blood, mucus or worms in the stool**
- **Black colored stools**
- **Severe abdominal or rectal pain**
- **Dry mouth**
- **Wrinkled skin**
- **Excessive thirst and little or no urination**

YES SEE DOCTOR

NO ↓

In a child or adult, has the diarrhea lasted 48 hours or more and/or is fever of 101°F or higher present?

YES SEE DOCTOR

NO ↓

Is the diarrhea occurring more than 8 times per day in an infant or chronically ill elderly adult? YES 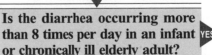 CALL DOCTOR

NO ↓

flowchart continued on next page

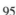

Diarrhea, continued

In a child or adult, are any medicines being taken (this includes regular medicines that the body may not be absorbing due to the diarrhea, or prescribed or over-the-counter ones that might be contributing to diarrhea)?

YES → CALL DOCTOR

NO

Did diarrhea come on during or shortly after returning from a trip to a foreign country?

YES → CALL DOCTOR

NO

USE SELF-CARE

Self-Care Tips

Steps to control diarrhea:

With more fluid than usual being flushed out of your body, dehydration is a potential problem, especially with infants and children, who have less fluid to spare than adults.

- The first course of action is to drink plenty of clear fluids. Even sucking on ice chips helps. Adults should have around 2 cups of fluid per hour (if vomiting isn't present). For children under 2, you should consult their doctor about amount and type of fluid. For children over 2, give up to 2 quarts of fluid per day (consult their doctor when in doubt or if they show any signs of dehydration, i.e., thirst, muscle cramps, delirium, weakness). Ready-made solutions such as Pedialyte and Lytren that restore fluids and minerals, available in most drug stores, are often recommended for children. They can also be used for adults.

- Other clear liquids to give include: Water, Jello (both in liquid and solid form), clear broths, sodas such as ginger ale, flat cola, 7-Up, Sprite, etc., weak tea with sugar, and sport drinks such as Gatorade.

- You can also make your own solution by mixing: 4 teaspoons of sugar and 1 teaspoon of salt with 1 quart (4 cups) of water.

- Avoid very hot and very cold liquids, however, since they can stimulate the colon. Also, avoid drinking apple juice. It sometimes worsens diarrhea, especially in children. Don't drink milk at this time, either. It also worsens diarrhea.

- Eat little or no solid food for the first few days. (Jello is okay - it counts as a clear liquid).

- When diarrhea is waning, following a B.R.A.T. diet: Bananas (ripe), rice, applesauce, and toast. These foods tend to be constipating, and should be the first things you eat after a bout of diarrhea.

- Once the diarrhea has subsided, eat small amounts of semi-soft foods, like cooked potatoes. Stay away from dairy products and foods that contain a lot of protein such as meat.

- Don't eat high-fiber foods like whole-grain breads and bran cereals.

- Avoid eating raw fruits and vegetables and fried foods or drinking coffee, all of which are hard on your digestive tract.

- Limit physical activity until bowel activity returns to normal.

- Try Kaopectate, Immodium AD or other non-prescription remedies containing bismuth, such as Pepto-Bismol. *[Note: Do not give aspirin or any medication containing salicylates to anyone 19 years of age or younger unless directed by a physician, due to its association with Reye's Syndrome, a potentially fatal condition.]* Follow package directions to the letter. Don't take these right away, though. Letting the diarrhea run its course for at least 12 hours allows the body to rid itself of whatever is causing the diarrhea.

- Always make sure to wash your hands after going to the toilet and before preparing food, especially when you have diarrhea which results from an infection in the GI tract. Don't share towels with others. Use disposable paper towels to dry your hands.

Flatulence

Flatulence may be perfectly natural and something that everyone gets, but if you have more than your share, it's a major annoyance.

Where does all that gas come from, anyway? Often, it comes from swallowing air. It's also generated by intestinal bacteria that produce carbon dioxide and hydrogen (both odorless, by the way) in the course of breaking down carbohydrates and proteins in the food you eat. The minute quantities of other, more pungent gases gives flatus its characteristic odor. Eating certain foods, like peas, beans, and certain grains produces noticeably more gas than eating other foods. All roughages in the diet will produce flatulence. A high roughage diet, especially, will do this. When increasing dietary fiber in your diet, do so gradually. This will lessen the increase of flatus. Gas may signal a variety of other problems worth looking into:

- Lactose intolerance (inability to properly digest milk, cheese, and other dairy products).
- Bacterial overgrowth in the intestines (often caused by certain antibiotics).
- Abnormal muscle contraction in the colon.

Questions To Ask

Is the flatulence accompanied by severe steady pain in the upper abdomen, nausea and vomiting, or yellowing of the skin or eyes? YES → SEE DOCTOR

NO ↓

Has the flatulence occurred only after taking a prescribed antibiotic? YES → CALL DOCTOR

NO ↓

USE SELF-CARE

Self-Care Tips

Common sense says eliminating food items that often cause gas (or eating them in small quantities) can go a long way toward reducing excess flatulence. Well-known offenders include:

- Apples
- Apricots
- Beans (dried, cooked)
- Bran
- Broccoli
- Brussels sprouts
- Cabbage
- Carrots
- Cauliflower
- Dairy products (for persons allergic to lactose)
- Eggplant
- Nuts
- Onions
- Peaches
- Pears
- Popcorn
- Prunes
- Raisins
- Sorbitol
- Soybean

[Note: Eliminate or go easy on only the foods that affect you personally. With the exception of sorbitol, these foods listed provide nutrients, so should not be cut out altogether.]

- Keep a list of all of the foods you eat for a few days and note when and the number of times you have gas. If you notice that you have excess gas after drinking milk, for example, try cutting down on it or eliminate it from your diet. See if the flatulence persists. Do the same for other suspecting foods.
- If you are lactose-intolerant use lactose-reduced dairy foods or add an over-the-counter lactose-enzyme product such as Lactaid. These can be drops or tablets that you add to or consume with dairy products to help you digest the lactose they contain.
- Avoid swallowing air at mealtimes.
- The medication simethicone may help reduce flatulence by dispersing gas pockets (and preventing more from forming). It has no known side effects. Simethicone is available by prescription as well as over-the-counter under the brand name Mylicon.
- An over-the-counter product called BEAN-O may curb flatulence caused by eating some foods.

Heartburn

Heartburn has nothing to do with the heart. Rather, it involves the esophagus (the tube that connects the throat to the stomach), and the stomach itself. The esophagus passes behind the breastbone alongside the heart, so the inflammation or irritation that takes place there feels like a burning sensation in the heart.

What causes this irritation? Gastric acids from the stomach splash back up into the lower portion of the esophagus, causing pain. The digestive acids don't harm the stomach, thanks to its protective coating, but the esophagus has no such armor which results in discomfort. The most common heartburn triggers are:

- Taking aspirin, ibuprofen, naproxen sodium, arthritis medicine, or cortisone.
- Eating heavy meals or eating rapidly.
- Eating foods like chocolate, garlic, onions, peppermint, tomatoes or citrus fruits.
- Lying down after a meal.
- Smoking after eating.
- Drinking coffee (regular or decaffeinated).
- Drinking alcohol.
- Being very overweight.
- Wearing tight clothing.
- Pregnancy.
- Swallowing too much air.
- Stress.
- A weakened or malfunctioning valve between the esophagus and the stomach.
- A bulging of the upper part of the stomach through the diaphragm. This is called gastroesophageal reflux disease (GERD). It was commonly termed hiatal hernia.

Questions to Ask

Do you have any of the following?
- **A tightness in your chest which radiates to the neck, jaw or arm**
- **Sweating or shortness of breath**
- **Nausea**
- **Discomfort that gets worse with exertion**

YES → SEEK EMERGENCY CARE

NO ↓

flowchart continued in next column

Are you vomiting black or red-colored material? YES → SEEK EMERGENCY CARE

NO ↓

Are your stools tar-like and black in color? YES → SEE DOCTOR

NO ↓

Do you also have pain that goes through to your back or a gripping pain in the upper abdomen? YES → SEE DOCTOR

NO ↓

Are you having a hard time swallowing? YES → CALL DOCTOR

NO ↓

Has the heartburn occurred often over 3 days? YES → CALL DOCTOR

NO ↓

USE SELF-CARE

Self-Care Tips

Treatment consists of avoiding as many contributing factors as possible, plus the following:

- Sit straight, and stand up or walk around whenever you can. Bending over or lying down after eating makes it too easy for gastric secretions to move up to the esophagus.
- If heartburn bothers you at night, raise the head of the bed slightly. (Example: Put the head of your bed up on 6 inch blocks, or buy a wedge especially made for putting between the mattress and box spring).
- Lose weight if you are overweight.
- Avoid wearing tight-fitting garments around the abdomen. (Example: Girdle).
- Eat small meals. Limit alcohol.
- Limit foods and drinks that contain air. (Example: Baked goods, waffles, whipped cream, carbonated beverages).
- Don't drink through straws or bottles with narrow mouths.

Heartburn, continued

- ☐ Don't eat for 2 to 3 hours before bedtime.
- ☐ If other treatments fail:
  - Take an antacid. They coat your stomach and neutralize acids. For example, take 1 to 2 tablespoons of a non-absorbable liquid antacid such as magnesium hydroxide every 2 to 4 hours or ones that come in tablet form such as Tums.
  - If antacids don't bring relief take an over-the-counter acid controller, (examples - Pepcid AC and Tagamet HB.) These not only relieve heartburn but can prevent it. *[Note: Read label before taking antacids or acid controllers. If you have questions check with your doctor.]*
- ☐ Don't take baking soda. It may neutralize stomach acid at first, but when its effects wear off, the acid comes back to a greater degree causing severe gastric acid rebound.
- ☐ Don't smoke. It promotes heartburn.
- ☐ If you do take aspirin, ibuprofen, naproxen sodium, or arthritis medicines, take them with food.

[Note: Call your doctor if you find no relief from self-care tips.]

Vomiting and Nausea

Vomiting is when you throw up what is in your stomach. Nausea is when you feel like you're going to throw up. Common causes of nausea and vomiting are:

- ☐ Viruses in the intestines (You can get diarrhea, too).
- ☐ Morning sickness in pregnant women.
- ☐ Some medications.
- ☐ Spoiled food.
- ☐ Eating or drinking too much.

Some serious problems cause vomiting, too. These include:

- ☐ Appendicitis.
- ☐ Brain tumors.
- ☐ Acute glaucoma.
- ☐ Stomach ulcers.
- ☐ Hepatitis - inflammation of the liver.
- ☐ Meningitis - inflammation of membranes that cover the brain and spinal cord.

Questions to Ask

Do you have any of these problems along with the vomiting?
- **Stiff neck, fever and headache**
- **Black or bloody vomit**
- **Very bad pain in and around one eye**
- **Blurry eyesight**
- **A head injury that happened a short time ago**

YES SEEK EMERGENCY CARE

NO

Dehydration is when your body loses too much water. Do you have any of these signs of dehydration?
- **Feeling confused**
- **Very little or no urine**
- **Sunken eyes**
- **Skin that is wrinkled or sags**

YES SEEK EMERGENCY CARE

NO

Do you have these symptoms with vomiting?
- **Fever and shaking chills**
- **Pain in one or both sides of your lower back**

YES SEEK EMERGENCY CARE

NO

Do you have very bad stomach pain? Does it last for more than 2 hours? Does it keep hurting even after you throw up?

YES SEE DOCTOR

NO

Do the whites of your eyes or your skin look yellow?

YES SEE DOCTOR

NO

Do you have these problems?
- **Burning or stinging feeling when you pass urine**
- **Passing urine a lot more often than usual**
- **Bloody or cloudy urine**
- **Pain in your abdomen or over your bladder**

YES SEE DOCTOR

NO

flowchart continued on next page

Vomiting & Nausea, continued

Have you been throwing up for more than 12 hours without getting better? **YES** → CALL DOCTOR

NO

In a small child, has the vomiting lasted 2 to 6 hours? **YES** → CALL DOCTOR

NO

Are you throwing up medicine that is necessary for you to take? (Birth control pills and high blood pressure pills are examples). **YES** → CALL DOCTOR

NO

USE SELF-CARE

Self-Care Tips

- Don't eat solid food until you stop throwing up.
- Drink clear liquids at room temperature (not too cold or too hot). Take small sips. Drink only 1 to 2 ounces at a time. Water, "flat" cola, and ginger ale are good. Stir any carbonated beverages to get all the bubbles out before sipping them. Don't drink alcohol. Suck on ice chips if nothing else will go down.
- After you stop throwing up, you can go from clear liquid foods like Jell-O (any color but red) and broth to liquids like milk. Try soft foods after that, such as bananas, rice, applesauce and toast.
- Over-the-counter medications like Emetrol may help.
- Don't smoke.
- Don't take aspirin.
- Call your doctor if you don't get better or if the vomiting comes back.

chapter 14

MUSCLE & BONE PROBLEMS

Backaches

Most backaches come from strained muscles in the lower back. Other causes include back injuries such as a slipped or herniated disc, arthritis, osteoporosis, and urinary tract infections. The goals of treatment are to treat the cause of the backache, relieve the pain, promote healing and avoid re-injury.

Improper lifting causes a lot of backaches. Here are some lifting "dos and don'ts" to help you avoid straining your back.

Dos

- ▱ Wear good shoes with low heels, not sandals or high heels.
- ▱ Stand close to the thing you want to lift.
- ▱ Plant your feet squarely, shoulder width apart.
- ▱ Bend at the knees, not at the waist. Keep your knees bent as you lift.
- ▱ Pull in your stomach and rear-end. Keep your back as straight as you can.
- ▱ Hold the object close to your body.
- ▱ Lift slowly. Let your legs carry the weight.
- ▱ Get help or use a dolly to move something that is too big or very heavy.

Don'ts

- ▱ Don't lift if your back hurts.
- ▱ Don't lift if you have a history of back trouble.
- ▱ Don't lift something that's too heavy.
- ▱ Don't lift heavy things over your head. Don't lift anything heavy if you're not steady on your feet.
- ▱ Don't bend at the waist to pick something up.
- ▱ Don't arch your back when you lift or carry.
- ▱ Don't lift too fast or with a jerk.
- ▱ Don't twist your back when you are holding something. Turn your whole body, from head to toe.

- ▱ Don't lift something heavy with one hand and something light with the other. Balance the load.
- ▱ Don't try to lift one thing while you hold something else. For example, don't try to pick up a child while you are holding a grocery bag. Put the bag down, or lift the bag and the child at the same time.

Questions to Ask

Is the back pain <u>extreme</u> and felt across the upper back (not just on one side) and did it come on suddenly (within about fifteen minutes) with no apparent reason such as an injury or back strain? *[Note: These may be symptoms of a dissecting aortic aneurysm.]*

NO

Did the back pain start inside your chest and move to the upper back? *[Note: You may be having a heart attack. The pain may be dull and you may not feel it in the chest at all.]*

NO

Was the back pain sudden with a cracking sound?

NO

Did the pain come after a recent fall, injury, or violent movement to the back and are you having a hard time moving your arm or leg? Do you also have numbness or tingling in your legs, feet, toes, arms or hands and/or loss of bladder or bowel control?

NO

flowchart continued on next page

Backaches, continued

Did the pain come on all of a sudden after being in a wheelchair or a long stay in bed, or are you over 60 years old? **YES** SEE DOCTOR

NO

Is the pain severe, (but not a result from a fall or injury to the back), and has it lasted for more than five to seven days or is there also a sense of weakness, numbness or tingling in the feet or toes? **YES** SEE DOCTOR

NO

Does the pain travel down the leg(s) below the knee? **YES** SEE DOCTOR

NO

Does the pain get worse with movement, coughing, sneezing, lifting or straining or does it come with a loss of bowel and/or bladder control? **YES** SEE DOCTOR

NO

Are any of the following also present?
- **Difficulty in urinating such as pain, burning or itching**
- **Increased urge or frequency**
- **Foul smelling urine or blood in the urine**
- **Fever and shaking chills**
- **Abdominal pain**

YES SEE DOCTOR

NO

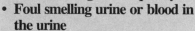
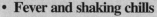

Is the pain felt on one side of the small of your back, just above your waist and do you feel sick and have a fever of 101°F or higher? **YES** SEE DOCTOR

NO

flowchart continued in next column

Do you also have any of the following?
- **Joint stiffness and pain**
- **Redness, heat or swelling in affected joints**
- **Cracking or grating sounds with joint movement**

YES SEE DOCTOR

NO

 USE SELF-CARE

Self-Care Tips
Activity

Continue your regular activities as much as you can. Rest the back if you must, but don't rest in bed more than 2-3 days, even if your back hurts a lot. Your back muscles can get weak if you don't use them or if you stay in bed longer than 3 days. To make the most of rest:

- Get comfortable when you are lying, standing, and sitting. For example, when you lie on your back, keep your upper back flat, but your hips and knees bent. Keep your feet flat on the bed. Tip your hips down and up until you find the best spot.
- Put a pillow under your knees or lie on your side with your knees bent. This will take pressure off your lower back.
- When you get up from bed, move slowly, roll on your side, and swing your legs to the floor. Push off the bed with your arms.

Cold Treatment

Cold helps with bruises and swelling. For the first 48 hours after back symptoms start, apply a cold pack (or bag of ice) to the painful area. Lie on your back with your knees bent, and put the cold pack under your lower back. Do this for 5-10 minutes at a time, several times a day.

Backaches, continued

Heat Treatment

Heat makes blood flow, which helps healing. But don't use heat on a back strain until 48 or more hours after back symptoms start. If used sooner, heat can make the pain and swelling worse. Use a moist heating pad, a hot-water bottle, hot compresses, a hot tub, hot baths, or hot showers. Use heat for 10 minutes at a time. Do this several times a day. Be careful not to burn yourself.

Massage

Massage won't cure a backache, but it can loosen tight muscles.

Braces or Corsets

Braces and corsets support your back and keep you from moving it too much. They do what strong back muscles do, but they won't make your back stronger.

Relieve the Pain

Take aspirin, ibuprofen, or naproxen sodium for pain. *[Note: Do not give aspirin or any medication containing salicylates to anyone 19 years of age or younger, unless directed by a physician, due to its association with Reye's Syndrome, a potentially fatal condition.]* Acetaminophen will help with pain, but not swelling.

Don't "overdo it" after taking a pain killer. You can hurt your back more, and then it will take longer to heal.

More Tips

- Try some mild stretching exercises (in the morning and afternoon) to make your stomach and back muscles stronger. Always ask your doctor before starting an exercise program.
- Don't sit in one place longer than you need to. It strains your lower back.
- Sleep on a firm mattress.
- Never sleep on your stomach. Sleep on your back or side, with your knees bent.

- If your back pain is chronic or doesn't get better on its own, see your doctor. He or she can evaluate your needs. A referral may be given to a physical therapist, a physiatrist (a physical therapy doctor), or a chiropractor.

Broken Bones

You may think that the body's 206 bones are as dry and lifeless as a dead tree branch. Not so. Bones are made up of living tissue. New bone is added and old bone is broken down daily. This nonstop process continues from our first year until we hit 35 years. At about this age, our bones gradually start to thin as the building process slows down.

Bones break when stressed. An arm, leg or finger, like a tree limb twisted in the wrong direction, hit too hard or crushed by accident, can splinter and snap.

There are different kinds of broken bones:
- Simple or closed fractures - The broken bone is not visible through the skin nor is there a skin wound near the fracture site. An example of this is a greenstick fracture. It is called this because the X-ray resembles the pattern of a very young splintered green twig.
- Compound or open fracture - A bone may separate partially or completely and a skin wound is also present. The bone can protrude through the skin or the skin has been cut due to the injury.

Bones in children are more pliable and resilient than those in adults. In most cases, children's bones are still growing, especially the long bones of their arms and legs. Damage to the ends of these bones should be monitored carefully because of the risk of stunting the bone's growth.

Broken Bones, continued

Bones in some senior citizens become dangerously thin with age. Many postmenopausal women and some elderly men suffer from osteoporosis, a condition in which the bones after age 35 begin losing their ability to absorb calcium from the blood. The bones in people with osteoporosis become brittle and break easily. The female hormone estrogen protects women from osteoporosis until they pass through menopause. Estrogen Replacement Therapy (ERT) can help after menopause.

Broken bones need immediate treatment. Not only are they intensely painful, but unless properly cared for, broken bones may cause future deformities and limited movement.

Prevention

Make sure you and your child wear appropriate protective gear, such as shoulder pads, knee pads, and a helmet, etc., during sporting and recreation events.

Check that everyone in the car is wearing a seat belt. Don't start the engine until everyone has buckled up.

If you or your child likes to roller-blade, these tips may prevent injury:

- ☐ Always wear a helmet, elbow and knee pads and wrist guards.
- ☐ Skate on smooth, paved surfaces.
- ☐ Avoid skating at night.
- ☐ Learn how to stop.

If you are a postmenopausal woman, talk to your physician about Estrogen Replacement Therapy (ERT), alendronate sodium (Fosamax), calcitonin and:

- ☐ Exercise. Moderate, weight-bearing exercise such as walking, aerobics and dancing increases bone mass.
- ☐ Eat calcium-rich foods such as low-fat milk products, sardines, broccoli and calcium-fortified foods, such as juices, cereals and breads.
- ☐ Take calcium supplements if necessary.
- ☐ If you smoke, quit. If you drink, limit the amount.

Questions to Ask

Does the person have an injury to the head, neck, and/or back?

NO

Does the victim have severe bleeding and/or an open fracture?

NO

Is the person showing these signs of shock:
- **Fainting**
- **Sweating, dizziness, increased thirst, rapid, weak pulse rate**
- **Cold, pale and clammy skin**

NO

Does the person have:
- **A broken bone in the pelvis or thigh**
- **Cold, blue skin under the fracture**
- **Numbness below the fracture**

NO

If a rib is cracked, is the person also suffering shortness of breath? Is there any deformity at the fracture site?

NO

Is the pain so severe the person is unable to bear weight on the injured limb and/or is there a lot of bruising around the injury?

NO

104

Self-Care Tips

All broken bones require a doctor's attention. Do not try to set a broken bone yourself or try to push a protruding bone back under the skin. However, you may need to immobilize the injured limb until you get medical attention.

- A splint is a good way to immobilize the affected area, reduce pain and prevent shock.
  - Effective splints can be made from rolled-up newspapers and magazines, an umbrella, a stick, a cane and rolled up blankets. Place this type of item around the injury and gently hold it in place with a necktie, strip of cloth or belt. The general rule is to splint a joint above and below the fracture.
  - Lightly tape or tie an injured leg to the uninjured one, putting padding between the legs, if possible. Tape an injured arm to the chest, if the elbow is bent, or to the side if the elbow is straight, placing padding between the body and the arm.
  - For a broken arm, make a sling out of a triangular piece of cloth. Place the forearm in it and tie the ends around the neck so the arm is resting at a 90° angle.
  - Check the pulse in the splinted limb. If you cannot find it, the splint is too tight and must be loosened at once.
  - Check for swelling, numbness, tingling or a blue tinge to the skin. Any of these signs indicate the splint is too tight and must be immediately loosened to prevent permanent injury.
  - Keep the person quiet to avoid moving the injured area.
- Apply ice to the injured area to help reduce swelling and inflammation.
- Take aspirin, (avoid if bleeding) ibuprofen or naproxen sodium to reduce pain and swelling. Acetaminophen will help the pain, but not the swelling. [Note: Do not give aspirin or any medication containing salicylates to anyone 19 years of age or younger, unless directed by a physician, due to its association with Reye's Syndrome, a potentially fatal condition.]

Shoulder & Neck Pain

Shoulder and neck pain is a common condition. Driving a golf ball, cleaning windows or reaching for a jar can strain and injure shoulder muscles and tendons, especially in people who are out of condition. Fortunately, this discomfort rarely suggests a serious condition. Causes of shoulder and neck pain include:

- Poor posture and/or unnatural sleeping positions.
- Sleeping on a soft mattress can give you a stiff neck the next morning.
- Tension and stress. When you feel tense, the muscles around your neck can go into spasms.
- Tendinitis, inflammation of a tendon, the cord-like tissue that connects muscles to bone. Left untreated, tendinitis can turn into "frozen shoulder", a stiff, painful condition that may limit your ability to use your shoulder.
- Bursitis, an inflammation of the sac (bursa) that encases the shoulder joint. Bursitis can be caused by injury, infection, overuse, arthritis or gout.
- Osteoarthritis. Unlike rheumatoid arthritis, osteoarthritis develops from normal wear-and-tear of the joints as we age or from repeated injuries. Aging can cause the joints to wear out, producing bony spurs that can press on nerves and cause pain.
- Accidents and falls. Collarbones can break after falls or auto accidents.
- Motor vehicle accidents. You can develop a whiplash injury when your vehicle is hit from behind.
- Pinched nerve. Arthritis or an injury to your neck can pinch a nerve in your neck. Pain from a pinched nerve usually runs down the arm and one side only.

Sometimes shoulder and neck pain signal serious medical problems, especially with other symptoms such as stiff neck, sudden and severe headache, dizziness, chest pain or pressure, and/or loss of consciousness.

Shoulder & Neck Pain, continued

Prevention

- Stretching and strengthening routines, especially before exercising, helps prevent tendinitis. So can using the right equipment and following the proper technique.
- Avoid injuries to the shoulder by wearing seat belts in cars and trucks and using protective gear during sporting events.
- Avoid vigorous exercise unless you are fit. If you are out of condition, start to strengthen your muscles gradually and slowly increase exercise intensity.
- Don't sleep on your stomach. You are likely to twist your neck in this position.
- Sleep on a firm mattress. Use a feather, polyester or special neck (cervical) pillow. Use a thinner pillow or none at all if you have pain when you wake up.

Keep the muscles in your shoulders strong and flexible to prevent injury. These exercises can help:

- Stretch the back of your shoulder by reaching with one arm under your chin and across the opposite shoulder, gently push the arm toward your collarbone with the other hand. Hold for 15 seconds. Repeat five times, then switch sides.
- Raise one arm and bend it behind your head to touch the opposite shoulder. Use the other hand to gently pull the elbow toward the opposite shoulder. Hold for 15 seconds. Repeat five times, then switch sides.
- Holding light weights, lift your arms out horizontally and slightly forward. Keeping your thumbs toward the floor, slowly lower your arms halfway, then return to shoulder level. Repeat ten times.
- Sit straight in a chair. Flex your neck slowly forward and try to touch your chin to your chest. Hold for 10 seconds and go back to the starting position. Repeat five times.

- Sit straight in a chair. Look straight ahead. Slowly tilt your head to the right, trying to touch your right ear to your right shoulder. Do not raise your shoulder to meet your ear. Hold for 10 seconds and straighten your head. Repeat five times on this side and then on your left side.

Questions to Ask

Along with the shoulder and neck pain are you:
- **Feeling pressure in your chest, especially on the left side?**
- **Short of breath or having trouble breathing?**
- **Nauseous and/or vomiting?**
- **Sweating?**
- **Anxious?**
- **Having irregular heartbeats?**

YES → SEEK EMERGENCY CARE

NO ↓

Did you experience a serious injury that caused shoulder and/or neck pain that is not going away and/or is getting worse?

YES → SEEK EMERGENCY CARE

NO ↓

Do you have a stiff neck along with a severe headache, fever, nausea and vomiting?

YES → SEEK EMERGENCY CARE

NO ↓

Do you have any of the following?
- **Severe or persistent pain, swelling, spasms or a deformity in your shoulder?**
- **A shoulder that is painful and stiff with reduced ability to move it?**
- **Stabbing pain, numbness or tingling?**
- **Pain, tenderness and limited motion in the shoulder?**

YES → SEE DOCTOR

NO ↓

flowchart continued on next page

Shoulder & Neck Pain, continued

Is the shoulder pain severe or interfering with your sleep? Is the shoulder stiff in the morning, swollen, tender or hard to move?

YES — CALL DOCTOR

NO

USE SELF-CARE

Self-Care Tips

Unfortunately, no matter how careful people are, injuries do occur. Injured tendons, muscles and ligaments in any part of the body can take a long time to heal. Longer, in fact, than a broken bone. Don't ignore the aches and pains. Studies show that exercising before an injury has healed may not only worsen it, but may greatly increase the chance for re-injury.

Put the arm with the injured shoulder in a sling when you take the person to the doctor.

Treating Tendinitis - Taking over-the-counter pain relievers such as aspirin, ibuprofen or naproxen sodium eases the pain and reduces inflammation. Acetaminophen eases muscle soreness but does not help with inflammation. *[Note: Do not give aspirin or any medication containing salicylates to anyone 19 years of age or younger, unless directed by a physician, due to its association with Reye's Syndrome, a potentially fatal condition.]*

R.I.C.E. - Rest, ice, compression and elevation, is the accepted treatment for tendinitis. While the pain could linger for weeks, with the proper and immediate treatment, it usually disappears in a few days.

R Rest the injured shoulder. Rest prevents further inflammation, giving the tendon a chance to heal. Resume your activities only after the pain is completely gone.

I Ice the injured area as soon as possible. Immediately putting ice on the injury helps to speed recovery because it not only relieves pain, but also slows blood flow, reducing internal bleeding and swelling.
- Put ice cubes or crushed ice in a heavy plastic bag with a little water. You can also use a bag of frozen vegetables. Wrap the ice pack in a towel before placing it on the injured areas.
- Apply the ice pack to the injured shoulder for 10 to 20 minutes. Reapply it every two hours and for the next 48 hours during the times you are not sleeping.

C Compress the shoulder injury. Wear a sling to keep the shoulder from moving, to prevent further damage, and to remind yourself to take it easy.

E Elevate the shoulder whenever possible to further reduce the swelling.

The swelling is usually eased within 48 hours. Once the swelling is gone, apply heat to speed up healing, help relieve pain, relax muscles and reduce joint stiffness.
- Use a heating pad set on low or medium or a heat lamp for dry heat. Or, use a hot-water bottle, heat pack or hot, damp towel wrapped around the injured area for moist heat. *[Note: Damp heat should be no warmer than 105°F.]*
- Apply heat to the injured area for 20 to 30 minutes, two to three times a day.

Liniments and balms also relieve the discomfort of sore muscles. They provide a cooling or warming sensation. Although these ointments only mask the pain of sore muscles and do nothing to promote healing, massaging them into the shoulder increases blood flow to help relax the muscles.

Treating Bursitis - Prolonged use of a joint or arthritis can cause the pain and discomfort of bursitis. Fortunately, these flare-ups can be controlled by:
- Applying ice packs to the sore shoulders.
- Taking a hot shower, using a heat lamp, applying a hot compress or heating pad to the affected shoulder, or rubbing the area with a deep-heating liniment.

Shoulder & Neck Pain, continued

Treating Neck Pain from Whiplash Injuries or Pinched Nerves - Always see a doctor anytime your motor vehicle is hit from the rear because the accident can cause a whiplash injury. The recommended treatment for whiplash injuries usually consists of using hot and cold packs, massage, exercises, sometimes a neck brace and pain-relieving medications such as aspirin, acetaminophen, ibuprofen and naproxen sodium. Once your symptoms subside, you can resume normal activity.

After first checking with your doctor, you can ease neck discomfort by:

- Resting as much as possible by lying on your back.
- Using cold and hot packs. See how to use them in the above section on treating tendinitis.
- Improving your posture. When sitting, select a chair with a straight back and push your buttocks into the chair's back. When standing, pull in your chin and stomach.
- Using a cervical (neck) pillow or rolling a hand towel and placing it under your neck.
- Avoiding activities that may aggravate your injuries.
- Covering your neck with a scarf in cold weather.
- Practicing some of the stretching and strengthening exercises listed under the section on prevention on page 106.

Dealing with Arthritis and Osteoporosis - See the section on arthritis on page 165 and the section on osteoporosis on page 172 for information on these conditions.

Sports Injuries

Common sports injuries include twisted ankles, painful joints, and stiff, sore muscles. If you continue to exercise when injured further damage can leave you laid up for weeks or months. "Break a leg" means good luck only in the theater. Take care to avoid injury when exercising.

Prevention

Common sense can prevent many sports injuries. Some typical injuries and ways to prevent them are listed below. The top six are:

Knee injury - knees are very susceptible to injury.
- Avoid locking your knees.
- Do not bend knees past 90° when doing half knee bends.
- Avoid twisting knees by keeping feet flat as much as possible (during stretches).
- Use the softest surface available when you exercise.
- Wear proper shoes with soft, flexible soles.
- When jumping, land with knees bent.

Muscle soreness - a symptom of having worked out too hard or too long.
- Do warm-up exercises such as those that stretch the muscles before your activity, not only for vigorous activities such as running but even for less vigorous ones such as golf.
- Don't overdo it.
- In vigorous activities, go through a cool-down period. Spend five minutes doing the activity at a slower pace. For example, after a run, walk or walk/jog for five minutes so your pulse comes down gradually.

Blisters - due to poor fitting shoes or socks.
- Wear shoes and socks that fit well. (The widest area of your foot should match the widest area of the shoe. You should also be able to wiggle your toes with the shoe on in both a sitting and standing position). The inner seams of the shoe should not rub against areas of your feet.
- Wear preventive taping, if necessary.

Side stitch - sharp pain felt underneath the rib cage.
- Don't eat or drink two hours prior to exercise.
- Do proper breathing by raising abdominal muscles as you breathe in.
- Don't "work through pain". Stop activity, then walk slowly.

Sports Injuries, continued

Shin splints - mild to severe ache in front of the lower leg.
- ☐ Strengthen muscles in this region.
- ☐ Keep calves well stretched.
- ☐ When using an indoor track, don't always run in the same direction.

Achilles tendon pain - caused by a stretch, tear, or irritation to the tendon that connects the calf muscles to the back of the heel.
- ☐ Do warm-up stretching exercises before the activity. Stretch the Achilles' tendon area and hold that position. Don't bounce.
- ☐ Wear proper fitting shoes that provide shock absorption and stability.
- ☐ Avoid running shoes with a heel counter that is "too" high.
- ☐ Avoid running on hard surfaces like asphalt and concrete.
- ☐ Run on flat surfaces instead of up hill. Running up hill aggravates the stress put on the Achilles' tendon.

Questions To Ask

Do you have any of the following?
- **Numbness and inability to move the injured body part**
- **Noticeable deformity of the extremity**

YES → SEEK EMERGENCY CARE

NO

Are any of these problems present?
- **More than mild pain and swelling**
- **Blue discoloration of the skin**

YES → SEE DOCTOR

NO

 USE SELF-CARE

Self-Care Tips

At the first sign of serious discomfort or pain, stop what you're doing and apply R.I.C.E. - rest, ice, compression, and elevation. By following this easy-to-remember formula, you can avoid further injury and speed recovery.

R Rest the injured area for 24 to 48 hours.

I Ice the area for 5 to 20 minutes every hour for the first 48 to 72 hours, or until the area no longer looks or feels hot.

C Compress the area by wrapping it tightly with an elastic bandage for 30 minutes, then unwrap it for 15 minutes. Begin wrapping from the point farthest from the heart (distally) and wrap toward the center of the body (proximally). Repeat several times.

E Elevate the area to reduce swelling. Prop it up to keep it elevated while you sleep.

Also, doctors recommend taking aspirin, ibuprofen or naproxen sodium to reduce inflammation and pain. (Take these with food or milk to prevent stomach irritation). *[Note: Do not give aspirin or any medication containing salicylates to anyone 19 years of age or younger, unless directed by a physician, due to its association with Reye's Syndrome, a potentially fatal condition.]*

Once the injured area begins to heal, do M.S.A. techniques. M.S.A. stands for movement, strength, and alternate activities.

M Movement - Work at establishing a full range of motion as soon as possible after an injury. This will help maintain flexibility during healing and prevent the scar tissue formed by the injury from limiting future performance.

S Strength - Gradually strengthen the injured area once the inflammation is controlled and a range of motion is re-established.

A Alternate Activities - Do regular exercise using activities that do not strain the injured part. This should be started a few days after the injury, even though the injured part is still healing.

Sprains & Strains

Common causes for sprains and strains are falls, twisting a limb, sports injuries, and over-exertion. A sprain results from overstretching or tearing a ligament (fibrous tissue that connects bones), a tendon (tissue that attaches a muscle to a bone) or a muscle. A strain occurs when a muscle or tendon is overstretched or over-exerted. Both sprains and strains result in pain and swelling. The amount of pain and swelling depends on the extent of damage.

Prevention

Common sense can prevent many sprains and strains. General safety measures to prevent slips and falls:

- Clear porches and walkways of ice in winter weather.
- Wear shoes and boots with non-skid soles.
- Install sturdy hand rails on both sides of stairways.
- Use rubber mats or adhesive-backed strips in bathtubs and shower stalls. Installing a support bar is also recommended.
- Make sure light switches are located near all room entrances inside of the house and to entrances outside.
- Use a night light between the bedroom and bathroom or in the hallway at night.
- Keep stairways and foot traffic areas clear of shoes, toys, tools, and other clutter.
- Floor coverings should be kept skid-proof. Vinyl floors should be cleaned with non-skid wax.
- Carpeting should be secured to the floor. Area rugs should have non-skid backing.
- Be careful whenever you use a ladder. Make sure it is steady and long enough to reach the job without standing on the top three steps.

To prevent sprains and strains from sports injuries:

- Ease into any exercise program. Start off with activities of low intensity, frequency, and duration and build up gradually.
- Do warm-up exercises such as those that stretch the muscles before your activity, not only for vigorous activities, such as running, but even for less vigorous ones, such as golf. Don't bounce.

- Don't overdo it. If muscles or joints start to hurt, ease up.
- In vigorous activities, go through a cool-down period. Spend five minutes doing the activity at a slower pace. For example, after a run, walk or stroll for five minutes so your pulse comes down gradually.
- Wear proper-fitting shoes that provide shock absorption and stability. Wear shoes designed for the sports activity you are doing.

Also, see the dos and don'ts of proper lifting in the section, "Backaches," on page 101.

Treatment for sprains and strains will depend on the extent of damage done to the muscle, ligament, tendon, etc. Self-help measures may be all that are needed for mild injuries. Severe sprains may require medical treatment. Some sprains require a cast. Others may need surgery if the tissue affected is torn.

Questions To Ask

Did the strain or sprain occur with great force from a vehicle accident or fall from a high place?

NO

Do you have any of these signs?
- **A bone sticking out or bones in the injured part make a grating sound**
- **The injured body part looks crooked or the wrong shape**
- **A loss of feeling in the injured body part**
- **You can't move the injured body part or put weight on it**

NO

flowchart continued on next page

Sprains & Strains, continued

Does the skin around the injury turn blue and/or feel cold and numb?	YES	SEE DOCTOR

NO

Do you have any of these signs? • There is bad pain and swelling or the pain is getting worse • It hurts to press along the bone	YES	SEE DOCTOR

NO

USE SELF-CARE

Self-Care Tips

- Stop what you're doing. Then use R.I.C.E. (See R.I.C.E. under Self-Care Tips for Sports Injuries on page 109).
- Take aspirin or ibuprofen every four hours for pain and inflammation. (Take with food or milk to prevent stomach irritation). *[Note: Do not give aspirin or any medication containing salicylates to anyone 19 years of age or younger unless directed by a physician, due to its association with Reye's Syndrome, a potentially fatal condition.]*

Also note, for specific areas of the body:

- Remove rings immediately if you have sprained a finger or other part of your hand. (If swelling occurs, the rings may have to be cut off).
- Use crutches to speed the healing process for a badly sprained ankle. They will help you avoid putting weight on the ankle which could cause further damage.

Call your doctor if the sprain or strain does not improve after four days of self-care tips.

chapter 15

OTHER HEALTH PROBLEMS

Anemia

Are you tired and weak? Do the linings of your lower eyelids look pale? If so, you could be anemic. But what does that mean? It means that either your red blood cells or the amount of hemoglobin (oxygen-carrying protein) in your red blood cells is low.

Iron-deficiency anemia is the most common form of anemia. In the United States, 20 percent of all women of childbearing age have iron-deficiency anemia (compared to 2 percent of adult men). The primary cause is blood lost during menstruation. But eating too few iron-rich foods or not absorbing enough iron can make the problem worse. (The recommended daily allowance for iron ranges from 6 milligrams (infants) to 30 milligrams (pregnant women). Yet one government source found that females between 12 and 50 years old, those at highest risk for iron-deficiency anemia, get about half of what they need). Pregnancy, breast-feeding a baby, and blood loss from the gastrointestinal tract (either due to ulcers or cancer) can also deplete iron stores. Older persons who have poor diets, especially when they live alone, often have iron-deficiency anemia.

Folic-acid deficiency anemia, another type of anemia, occurs when folic-acid levels are low, usually due to inadequate dietary intake or faulty absorption. The need for this vitamin more than doubles during pregnancy.

Other less common forms of anemia include pernicious anemia (inability of the body to properly absorb vitamin B_{12}), sickle cell anemia (an inherited disorder), and thalassemia anemia (also inherited).

Alcohol, certain medicines, and some chronic diseases can also cause anemia.

Questions To Ask

Do you have blood in your stools or urine or have black, tar-like stools with these problems?
- **Light headedness**
- **Weakness**
- **Shortness of breath**
- **Severe abdominal pain**

YES SEEK EMERGENCY CARE

NO

Are you dizzy when you stand up or when you exert yourself? YES SEE DOCTOR

NO

Do you have ringing in your ears? YES SEE DOCTOR

NO

For women:
- **Do you have menstrual bleeding between periods?**
- **Has menstrual bleeding been heavy for several months?**
- **Do you normally bleed seven days or more every month?**
- **Do you suspect that you are pregnant?**

YES CALL DOCTOR

NO

Do symptoms of anemia (paleness, tiredness, listlessness and weakness) persist despite using self-care tips (listed below) for at least two weeks? YES CALL DOCTOR

NO

USE SELF-CARE

Self-Care Tips

The first step in treating iron-deficiency anemia is to pinpoint the cause. If it's due to a poor diet, you're in luck: Iron deficiency anemia is not only the most common form of anemia, it's the easiest to correct if it's due to being female or taking in inadequate amounts of certain foods. Folic acid vitamin supplements may also be necessary.

You may need to:

- ▭ Eat more food that are good sources of iron. Concentrate on green, leafy vegetables, lean, red meat, beef liver, poultry, fish, wheat germ, oysters, dried fruit, and iron-fortified cereals.
- ▭ Boost your iron absorption. Foods high in vitamin C, such as citrus fruits, tomatoes, and strawberries, help your body absorb iron from food. And red meat not only supplies a good amount of iron, it also increases absorption of iron from other food sources.
- ▭ Don't drink a lot of tea—it contains tannins, substances that can inhibit iron absorption. (Herbal tea is okay, though).
- ▭ Take an iron supplement. (Consult your physician for proper dosage). While iron is best absorbed when taken on an empty stomach, it can upset your stomach. Taking iron with meals is less upsetting to the stomach. *[Note: Recent research is suggesting that high levels of iron in the blood may increase the risk for heart attacks. Do check with your doctor before taking iron supplements.]*
- ▭ Avoid antacids, phosphates (which are found in soft drinks, beer, ice cream, etc.) and the food additive EDTA. These block iron absorption.

Chest Pain

Chest pain can come from a lot of things. These include:

- ▭ A heart attack.
- ▭ Lung problems like pneumonia, bronchitis, or an injury.

- ▭ A hiatal hernia - known in medical terms as gastroesophageal reflux disease (GERD).
- ▭ Heartburn.
- ▭ Shingles.
- ▭ A pulled muscle.
- ▭ Mitral valve prolapse. A common disorder, especially in women, in which the mitral valve of the heart fails to close properly. In most people, this is not a serious problem.
- ▭ Anxiety.
- ▭ Swallowing too much air.

How do you know when you need medical help for chest pain? It's not always easy to tell. If you're not sure why your chest hurts, it's best to check it out. Getting help for a heart attack or lung injury could save your life.

Questions to Ask

Is the chest pain accompanied by any of the following?
- **Pain that spreads (radiates) to the arm, neck or jaw**
- **Feeling of pressure, especially on the left side**
- **Shortness of breath or trouble breathing**
- **Nausea and/or vomiting**
- **Sweating**
- **Uneven pulse or heartbeat**
- **Sense of doom**

 YES → SEEK EMERGENCY CARE

NO ↓

Did the chest pain result from a serious injury? Does it hurt all the time and/or is it getting worse? YES → SEEK EMERGENCY CARE

NO ↓

Does the chest pain occur in a person who has had a recent operation or illness that has kept them in bed? YES → SEEK EMERGENCY CARE

 NO ↓

flowchart continued on next page

Chest Pain, continued

Does the chest pain occur in a person with a history of heart problems or in a person with angina and not respond to prescribed medicine? YES SEEK EMERGENCY CARE

NO

Is there trouble breathing along with the chest pain? Does it get worse when taking deep breaths or when you touch your chest or ribs? YES SEE DOCTOR

NO

Are one or more of the following present?
- Fever
- Cough with sputum of any color (pink, green, yellow, gray, etc.)

YES SEE DOCTOR

NO

Do you have any of these problems with the chest pain?
- Palpitations
- Light-headedness
- Dizziness, feeling faint
- Fatigue
- Anxiety
- A heart murmur heard by a health care provider

YES SEE DOCTOR

NO

Does the chest pain last longer than two days? YES SEE DOCTOR

NO

Is the chest pain accompanied by belching and/or a burning sensation in the upper abdomen? Does it come and go before, during, or after eating, and does it worsen when bending or lying down? YES SEE DOCTOR

NO

flowchart continued in next column

Do all of these conditions describe the chest pain?
- It's only on one side of the chest
- It's unaffected by breathing
- It's accompanied by a burning feeling and a skin rash at the pain site

YES CALL DOCTOR

NO

 USE SELF-CARE

Self-Care Tips

For chest pain that results from a pulled muscle or minor injury to the rib cage:

- Do not strain the muscle or ribs while pain is felt.
- Rest.
- Take a pain reliever such as aspirin, acetaminophen or ibuprofen. *[Note: Do not give aspirin or any medication containing salicylates to anyone 19 years of age or younger unless directed by a physician, due to its association with Reye's Syndrome, a potentially fatal condition.]*
- Do call your doctor, though, if the pain lasts longer than two days.

For chest pain associated with a hiatal hernia:

- Lose weight if you are overweight.
- Eat 5-6 frequent meals, instead of 3 meals a day.
- Do not eat large meals.
- Avoid tobacco, alcohol, coffee, spicy foods, peppermint, chocolate, citrus juices and carbonated beverages.
- If you have heartburn, take antacids after meals and before going to bed.
- Do not eat food or drink milk two hours before going to bed.
- Avoid bending over or lying down after eating.
- Do not wear tight clothing, tight belts, or girdles.
- Raise the head of your bed about 3 to 4 inches (40 degree angle), when you sleep.

Chest Pain, continued

For chest pain that results from anxiety and hyperventilation:

- ☐ Talk over the source of your anxiety with family, friends, and clergy. If this is not enough, you may need the help of a professional counselor or psychiatrist.
- ☐ When you hyperventilate, cover your mouth and nose with a paper bag. Breathe into the paper bag slowly and re-breathe the air. Do this in and out at least 10 times. Remove the bag and breathe normally a few minutes. Repeat breathing in and out of the paper bag as needed.
- ☐ Avoid using large amounts of aspirin or other salicylate-containing medicines. *[Note: Do not give aspirin or any medication containing salicylates to anyone 19 years of age or younger unless directed by a physician, due to its association with Reye's Syndrome, a potentially fatal condition.]*

For chest pain associated with mitral valve prolapse (MVP):

- ☐ Eat healthy foods. Avoid caffeine.
- ☐ After checking with your doctor, exercise regularly to improve cardiovascular fitness.
- ☐ Deal with and control stress and avoid anxiety-producing situations, if possible.
- ☐ Don't smoke.

Fatigue

Fatigue is feeling tired, drained of energy and exhausted. Fatigue makes it hard for you to do normal daily activities. Feelings of inadequacy, low motivation and little desire for sex can also be symptoms of fatigue. There are many causes of fatigue.

Possible physical causes that need medical care include:

- ☐ Chronic fatigue syndrome. The fatigue lasts for six months or more.
- ☐ Lupus (the systemic type).
- ☐ Multiple sclerosis.
- ☐ Low thyroid.
- ☐ Leukemia.

- ☐ Having the AIDS virus.
- ☐ Anemia.
- ☐ Alcohol or drug abuse.

Other physical causes include:

- ☐ PMS. (See page 141).
- ☐ Lack of sleep.
- ☐ Crash dieting and eating poorly which results in vitamin and mineral deficiencies.
- ☐ Migraine headaches.
- ☐ Side effects from allergies or chemical sensitivities.
- ☐ Living or working in hot, humid conditions.
- ☐ Prolonged effects of the flu or a bad cold.

Possible emotional causes:

- ☐ Burnout.
- ☐ Boredom.
- ☐ Change (facing a major life crisis or decision like divorce or retirement).
- ☐ Depression and/or anxiety.

Treatment

The first thing to do is find the cause(s) of the fatigue so you know what to treat. It is important to keep track of any other symptoms that take place with the fatigue, so both physical and emotional causes can be identified and dealt with. For example, iron supplements can help with the fatigue that results from iron-deficiency anemia.

Questions to Ask

Do any of these problems occur with the fatigue?
- **Chest pain or tightness**
- **Shortness of breath**
- **Loss of balance or weakness, especially in one part or one side of the body**
- **Thoughts of suicide**

YES → SEEK EMERGENCY CARE

NO

flowchart continued on next page

Fatigue, continued

Do you have any of these problems with the fatigue?
- Loss of weight or appetite
- Yellow skin and/or eyes (jaundice)
- Blurry or double vision
- Throwing up a lot
- Feeling anxious, and not being able to calm down

YES →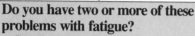

NO ↓

Do you have two or more of these problems with fatigue?
- Swollen lymph glands
- Sore throat
- Headache
- Painful swelling in the neck, armpit, or groin
- Fever
- Night sweats
- Excessive thirst and/or urination

YES → SEE DOCTOR

NO ↓

Do you have or have you had any of these problems?
- Arthritis or rheumatism for more than 3 months
- Fingers that get pale, numb or uncomfortable in the cold
- Mouth sores for more than two weeks
- Low blood counts from anemia, low white cell count or low platelet count
- A rash on your cheeks for more than one month
- Skin rash after being in the sun
- Pain for more than 2 days when taking deep breaths
- Fainting episode
- Seizure, convulsion or fit

YES → SEE DOCTOR

NO ↓

Did you start to feel fatigued after taking medicine?

YES → CALL DOCTOR

NO ↓

flowchart continued in next column

For women: Did the fatigue come with the onset of menopause, follow menopause or could you be pregnant?

YES → CALL DOCTOR

NO ↓

Has the fatigue lasted for more than two weeks and kept you from doing your usual activities for no apparent reason?

YES → CALL DOCTOR

NO ↓

 USE SELF-CARE

Self-Care Tips

Depending on the reasons for your fatigue, the following things may help restore your energy levels:

Eat healthier - Both extreme overeating and crash dieting can tax the body and lead to exhaustion. Skipping an important meal like breakfast or indulging in high fat and/or rich, sugary snacks are practically guaranteed to leave some people pooped. On the other hand, iron-rich foods, whole-grain breads and cereals and raw fruits and vegetables contain the nutrients your body needs to maintain your energy level. It may help to eat 5-6 light meals a day, instead of 3 large ones.

Get more exercise - Expending more energy can actually give you more energy, especially if you work at a sedentary job. Exercise also acts as a tranquilizer, counteracting emotionally induced anxiety or weariness. If you're feeling sluggish, try taking a brisk walk in the fresh air. It can renew your energy instantly.

Cool off - Working or playing in hot weather can drag you down, as can living or working in a warm, poorly ventilated environment. The solution to these problems is to rest in a cool, dry atmosphere as often as you can, drink plenty of liquids and open a window.

Fatigue, continued

Rest and relax - You don't need a book to tell you that getting a good night's sleep can put the spring back in your stride. But did you know that daily relaxation breaks can also restore your energy? Schedule your day to allow relaxation breaks, then practice deep breathing, meditation or yoga.

Change your routine - Nothing makes you feel stale faster than doing the same things over and over. Try to do something novel and interesting one or more times a day. If, on the other hand, you're on the go too much, set aside some time for peace and quiet.

Lighten your work load - Delegate tasks to others when you can, both at work and at home. Ask for help when you need it from family and friends or hire help if necessary.

Do something for yourself - Plan time to do things that meet only your needs, not just those of others.

Avoid too much caffeine and alcohol and don't use illegal drugs - These can trigger fatigue.

Fever

Elevated temperature isn't always a sign that something's wrong. Although 98.6°F has been considered normal for years, many healthy people walk around with a temperature a degree or so above or below average. A recent study has concluded that normal body temperature may range from 97°F to 100°F.

Body temperature even fluctuates throughout the day. It's usually lowest in the morning and highest in the late afternoon and evening. Where you measure your temperature also makes a difference. Rectal readings are usually more accurate and read a degree higher than oral readings.

Taking your temperature by mouth after you drink a hot liquid like soup or tea can mislead you into thinking you have a fever when you don't. Other factors that can temporarily affect your temperature include:

- ▢ Wearing too much clothing (if you're over-dressed enough to raise your body temperature).
- ▢ Exercise.
- ▢ Hot, humid weather.
- ▢ Hormones (increased progesterone levels increase body temperature, so women's basal body temperature increases following ovulation).

If you've ruled out other factors and your temperature is higher than 99°F, you might have a fever. If your temperature is higher than 100°F, you definitely have a fever.

Typically, in an adult, if having a fever causes no harm or discomfort, it may require no treatment. But if the fever is making you uncomfortable or goes over 104°F (102°F in the elderly) you should treat it.

Questions To Ask

Is the fever accompanied by any of the following?
- **Seizure**
- **Listlessness**
- **Abnormal breathing**
- **Stiff neck**
- **Excessive irritability**
- **Confusion**
- **Inability to be comforted**

YES → SEEK EMERGENCY CARE

NO ↓

Is the fever accompanied by any of the following?
- **Ear pain**
- **Persistent sore throat**
- **Vomiting**
- **Diarrhea**
- **Urinary pain, burning or frequency**

YES → SEE DOCTOR

NO ↓

Does the fever occur in a child less than 2 months old?

YES → SEE DOCTOR

NO ↓

flowchart continued on next page

117

Fever, continued

In an adult, does the fever exceed 104°F, (102°F in an elderly person), or has it lasted more than 4 days despite efforts to reduce the fever? YES SEE DOCTOR

NO

Has the person recently had surgery or does the person have a chronic illness, such as heart disease, lung disease, kidney disease, cancer or diabetes? YES CALL DOCTOR

NO

Does the fever occur in a baby less than 6 months old? YES CALL DOCTOR

NO

Has the fever done any of the following?
- **Gone away for more than 24 hours and then come back**
- **Come soon after a visit to a foreign country**
- **Come after having a DTP or MMR shot and is present with dizziness**

YES CALL DOCTOR

NO

In a child, does the fever over 101°F or (102°F rectally) without decreasing in 48 hours despite efforts to reduce the fever? YES CALL DOCTOR

NO

USE SELF-CARE

Self-Care Tips

▭ Drink fruit juice, water, and soft drinks.
▭ Take a sponge bath with warm (about 70°F) water. (Sponging with alcohol has no advantage and often makes people feel ill, because of alcohol's pungent odor).

▭ Take the appropriate dose of aspirin or acetaminophen for your age every 3 or 4 hours. *[Note: Do not give aspirin or any medication containing salicylates to a child 19 years of age or younger unless directed by a physician, due to its association with Reye's Syndrome, a potentially fatal condition.]*
▭ Get plenty of bed rest.
▭ Don't wear too many clothes or use too many blankets.
▭ Don't do heavy exercise.

Headaches

There are different kinds of headaches. The most common types are:

Tension or Muscular Headaches - You feel a dull ache in your forehead, above your ears, or at the back of your head. You get a tension headache when the muscles in your face, neck, or head get tight. This can happen when you:
▭ Don't get enough sleep.
▭ Feel "stressed out".
▭ Read.
▭ Do boring work.

Migraine Headaches - These happen when blood vessels in your head open too wide or close too tight. Women get migraines more than men. People in the same family often get them. A migraine headache makes your head throb. It feels like someone is hitting it with a big hammer. You may also get these symptoms:
▭ One side of your head hurts more than the other.
▭ You feel sick to your stomach or throw up.
▭ You see spots.
▭ Light hurts your eyes.
▭ Your ears ring.

Sinus Headaches - Your sinuses are behind your cheeks, around your eyes, and in your nose. You get a sinus headache when your sinuses swell up. Anybody can get a sinus headache. People with allergies like hay fever often get them.

Headaches, continued

A sinus headache makes your forehead, cheekbones, and nose hurt. It hurts more if you bend over or touch your face. You can get a sinus headache from:

- ▭ A cold.
- ▭ Allergies.
- ▭ Dirty or polluted air.
- ▭ Other breathing problems.

Headaches can also result from:

- ▭ A sensitivity to certain foods and drinks.
- ▭ Alcohol.
- ▭ Cigarette smoke.
- ▭ Exposure to chemicals and/or pollution.
- ▭ Poison.
- ▭ Side effects from some medications.

A headache can be a symptom of many health conditions too. Some of these are:

- ▭ Allergies.
- ▭ Depression.
- ▭ Fever.
- ▭ High blood pressure.
- ▭ Low blood sugar.
- ▭ Infections.
- ▭ Shingles.
- ▭ Dental problems.

Less often, a headache can be a symptom of a serious health problem that needs immediate medical attention. Examples are:

- ▭ Acute glaucoma.
- ▭ Stroke.
- ▭ Tumor, blood clot or ruptured blood vessel (aneurysm) in the brain.

To prevent headaches:

- ▭ Try to anticipate when pain will strike. Keep a headache journal that records when, where, and why headaches seem to occur.
- ▭ Note early symptoms and try to abort a headache in its earliest stages. Take pain medicine such as acetaminophen right away.

- ▭ Exercise regularly. This seems to keep some kinds of headaches at bay.
- ▭ Avoid foods and beverages known to trigger headaches in sensitive people. Try to figure out which foods and beverages affect you.

Particularly troublesome items may include:

- ▭ Alcoholic beverages, especially red wine.
- ▭ Aspartame (the artificial sweetener in NutraSweet™).
- ▭ Bananas. (If more than 1/2 banana a day.)
- ▭ Caffeine from coffee, tea, cola soft drinks, or some medications.
- ▭ Chocolate.
- ▭ Citrus fruits. (If more than 1/2 cup a day.)
- ▭ Cured meats such as frankfurters.
- ▭ Food additives such as monosodium glutamate (MSG).
- ▭ Hard cheeses such as aged cheddar or provolone.
- ▭ Nuts and peanut butter.
- ▭ Onions.
- ▭ Sour cream.
- ▭ Soy sauce.
- ▭ Vinegar.

Questions to Ask

Is the headache associated with any of the following?
- **A serious head injury**
- **A blow to the head that causes severe pain, enlarged pupils, vomiting, confusion or lethargy**
- **Loss of consciousness**

YES → SEEK EMERGENCY CARE

NO ↓

Is the headache associated with any of the following?
- **Pain in one eye**
- **Blurred vision**
- **Double vision**
- **Slurring of speech**
- **Mental confusion**
- **Personality change or problem in moving arms or legs**

YES → SEEK EMERGENCY CARE

NO ↓

flowchart continued on next page

Headaches, continued

Has the headache been occurring for more than 2-3 days, and increased in frequency and intensity?	YES SEEK EMERGENCY CARE

↓ NO

Is the headache associated with the following? • **Fever** • **Drowsiness** • **Nausea** • **Vomiting** • **Stiff neck**	YES SEEK EMERGENCY CARE

↓ NO

Has the headache come on suddenly, and does it hurt more than others you have had?	YES SEE DOCTOR

↓ NO

Has the headache occurred at the same time of day, week or month?	YES CALL DOCTOR

↓ NO

Have you noticed the headache only after taking newly prescribed or over-the-counter medicines?	YES CALL DOCTOR

↓ NO

USE SELF-CARE

Self-Care Tips

For on-the-spot headache relief:

- ☐ Take the recommended dose of acetaminophen, ibuprofen or naproxen sodium. Take it right away. (Pain killers work best when the headache starts). *Do not take aspirin unless it's O.K. with your doctor. [Note: Do not give aspirin or any medication containing salicylates to anyone 19 years of age or younger, unless directed by a physician, due to its association with Reye's Syndrome, a potentially fatal condition.]*
- ☐ Rest in a quiet, dark room with your eyes closed.
- ☐ Massage the base of your skull with your thumbs.
- ☐ Start under your ears and work back towards the center of your head. Also, massage both temples, your shoulders, neck and jaw gently.
- ☐ Take a warm bath or shower.
- ☐ Place a cold or warm washcloth, whichever feels better, over the area that aches. Or, put an ice pack on the back or top of the head if this brings relief.
- ☐ Relax. Try thinking of a calm, happy place.
- ☐ Breathe slowly and deeply.

Insomnia

Do you ever find yourself wide awake long after you go to bed at night? Well, you're not alone. An estimated 40 million Americans are bothered by insomnia. They either have trouble falling asleep at night, wake up in the middle of the night, or wake up too early and can't get back to sleep. And when they're not asleep, insomniacs worry about whether or not they'll be able to sleep. They are also irritable and feel fatigued during the day.

An occasional sleepless night is nothing to lose sleep over. But, if insomnia bothers you for three weeks or longer, it can be a real medical problem. Some medical problems that lead to insomnia include:

- ☐ Over-activity of the thyroid gland.
- ☐ Heart or lung conditions that cause shortness of breath when lying down.
- ☐ Depression, anxiety disorders.
- ☐ Allergies and early-morning wheezing.
- ☐ Any illness, injury or surgery that causes pain and/ or discomfort, such as arthritis, which interrupts sleep.
- ☐ Sexual problems (Example: Impotence).
- ☐ Hot flashes that interrupt sleep.
- ☐ Any disorder (urinary, gastrointestinal or neurological) that makes it necessary to urinate or have a bowel movement during the night.
- ☐ Side effects of certain medications (Examples: Decongestants, cortisone medications).

Insomnia, continued

Other things that lead to insomnia:

- Emotional stress.
- Too much noise when falling asleep. This includes a snoring partner.
- The use of stimulants such as caffeine from coffee, tea or colas, and stay awake pills such as NoDoz.
- A lack of physical exercise.
- Lack of a sex partner

Questions To Ask

Do you have trouble falling or staying asleep because of any of the following?
- **Pain or discomfort due to illness or injury**
- **The need to wake up to use the bathroom**

YES → CALL DOCTOR

NO

Has your sleep been disturbed since you began taking medication of any kind?

YES → CALL DOCTOR

NO

Do you still have trouble sleeping after 3 weeks, with or without self-care tips (see below)?

YES → CALL DOCTOR

NO

USE SELF-CARE

Self-Care Tips

Many old-fashioned remedies for sleeplessness work, and work well. Next time you find yourself unable to sleep, try these time-tested cures.

- Avoid caffeine in all forms after lunchtime. (Coffee, tea, chocolate, colas, and some other soft drinks contain this stimulant, as do certain over-the-counter and prescription medications. Check the labels for content).
- Avoid long naps during the day. (Naps decrease the quality of nighttime sleep).

- Avoid more than one or two servings of alcoholic beverages at dinner time and during the rest of the evening. Even though alcohol is a sedative, it can disrupt sleep. Always check with your doctor about using alcohol if you are taking medications.
- Have food items rich in the amino acid L-tryptophan such as milk, turkey or tuna fish before you go to bed. Eating foods with carbohydrates such as cereal, breads and fruits may help as well. (Do not, however, take L-tryptophan supplements).
- Take a nice, long, warm bath before bedtime. (This soothes and unwinds tense muscles, leaving you relaxed enough to fall asleep).
- Read a book or do some repetitive, tedious activity, like needlework. Try not to watch television or listen to the radio. These kinds of distractions may hold your attention and keep you awake.
- Make your bedroom as comfortable as possible. Create a quiet, dark atmosphere. Use clean, fresh sheets and pillows, and keep the room temperature comfortable (neither too warm nor too cool).
- Ban worry from the bedroom. Don't allow yourself to rehash the mistakes of the day as you toss and turn. You're off duty now. The idea is to associate your bed with sleep.
- Develop a regular bedtime routine. Locking or checking doors and windows, brushing your teeth, and reading before you turn in every night primes you for sleep.
- Count those sheep! Counting slowly is a soothing, hypnotic activity. By picturing repetitive, monotonous images, you may bore yourself to sleep.
- Try listening to recordings made especially to help promote sleep. Check local bookstores.
- Don't take over-the-counter sleeping pills or friends' or relatives' sleeping pills. Only take sleep medicine with your doctor's permission.

Snoring

Snoring is the sound heard when the airway is blocked during sleep. It can result from a number of things: obesity, enlarged tonsils and adenoids, deformities in the nasal passages, etc. Smoking, heavy drinking, overeating, especially before bedtime, and nasal allergies can lead to snoring by swelling the nasal passages and blocking the free flow of air. Also, persons who sleep on their backs are more likely to snore because the tongue falls back toward the throat and partly closes the airway. Nine out of ten snorers are men, and most of them are age 40 or over.

Snoring can be merely a nuisance or can be a signal of a serious health problem, sleep apnea, which might even require surgery. Sleep apnea is a condition where breathing is stopped for a time period of at least 10 seconds, but usually 20 to 30 seconds or even up to 1 or 2 minutes during sleep. It is more common in men than in women and typically affects men who are middle-aged and older. It can result from:

- An obstructed airway. This is more common as people age, especially those who are obese or who have smoked for many years.
- A central nervous system disorder such as a stroke, a brain tumor or even a viral brain infection.
- A chronic respiratory disease.

Questions To Ask

Do you notice the following signs of sleep apnea during your working hours:
- **Sleepiness or chronic daytime drowsiness**
- **Poor memory**
- **Lack of concentration**
- **Irritability**
- **Falling asleep while driving or working**
- **Loss of sex drive**
- **Headaches**

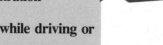

NO

flowchart continued in next column

Has someone else noticed that breathing has stopped for 10 seconds or longer (sleep apnea) in the midst of snoring? YES / SEE DOCTOR

NO

Has snoring persisted despite using the self-care tips below? YES / CALL DOCTOR

NO

 USE SELF-CARE

Self-Care Tips

- Sleep on your side. Prop an extra pillow behind your back so you won't roll over. Try sleeping on a narrow sofa for a few nights to get accustomed to staying on your side.
- Sew a large marble or tennis ball into a pocket on the back of your pajamas. The discomfort it causes will remind you to sleep on your side.
- If you must sleep on your back, raise the head of the bed by putting bricks or blocks between the mattress and box springs. Or buy a wedge especially made to be placed between the mattress and box spring to elevate the head section. Elevating the head prevents the tongue from falling against the back of the throat.
- If you are heavy, lose weight. Excess fatty tissue in the throat can cause snoring.
- Don't drink alcohol or eat a heavy meal within 3 hours before bedtime. For some reason, both seem to foster snoring.
- If necessary, take an antihistamine or decongestant before retiring to relieve nasal congestion (which can also contribute to snoring). *[Note: Older men should check with their doctor before taking decongestants. Decongestants that have ephendrine can give older men urinary problems.]*
- Get rid of allergens in the bedroom such as dust, down filled (feathered) pillows and bed linen (this may also relieve nasal congestion).
- Try over-the-counter "nasal strips". These keep the nostrils open and lift them up, keeping nasal passages unobstructed.

Urinary Tract Infections (UTIs)

About 1 out of 5 women will get a urinary tract infection (UTI) in her life. Some women get lots of UTIs. Men get UTIs, too, but not as often.

What is the urinary tract? Your urinary tract is made up of these parts:
- Kidneys.
- Bladder.
- Ureters (tubes that connect the kidneys to the bladder).
- Urethra (the tube through which urine is passed).

How do we get UTIs? Usually, bacteria get in the urethra and go to the bladder. They grow in the bladder and move to other parts of the urinary tract.

Bacteria can get into a woman's urethra during sex. You should go to the bathroom right after sex to flush the bacteria out. Women who use a diaphragm for birth control have twice the risk of getting a UTI. Changes that happen when you get pregnant and after menopause can also make you prone to UTIs.

Also, any irritation to the opening of the urethra can lead to bladder infections. If you have signs of a vaginal infection, (a discharge, foul odor, etc.) get treatment for it to help prevent a bladder infection.

Some people are born with urinary tract problems that help them get UTIs. Anything that keeps you from passing urine freely can lead to UTIs. Kidney stones or an enlarged prostate gland are two examples. You are also more likely to get a UTI if you have had UTIs before.

Sometimes you don't even know you have a UTI. Most often you will have symptoms, though. They come suddenly, with no warning. Here are some of them:
- A strong need to go to the bathroom.
- Going to the bathroom more often than usual.
- A sharp pain or burning in the urethra when you pass urine.
- Blood in the urine.
- Feeling like your bladder is still full after you pass urine.
- Soreness in your belly, back, or sides.
- Chills, fever, sick stomach, throwing up.

See a doctor if you have any of these symptoms. A UTI can be serious if you don't treat it. The doctor will test a sample of your urine to find the problem. An antibiotic to treat the infection and pain relievers (if necessary) are the usual course of treatment.

Prevention

Here are some things you can do to keep from getting UTIs:
- If you're a woman, wipe from front to back after using the toilet. This keeps bacteria away from the urethra.
- Drink plenty of liquids to flush bacteria out of your system. Drink fruit juices, especially cranberry juice.
- Empty your bladder as soon as you feel the urge. Don't give bacteria a chance to grow.
- Drink a glass of water before you have sex. Go to the bathroom as soon as you can after sex, even if you don't feel the urge.
- If you use a lubricant when you have sex, use a water-soluble lubricant like K-Y Jelly
- Wear cotton underpants. Bacteria like a warm, wet place. Cotton helps keep you cool and dry because it lets air flow through.
- Don't take bubble baths if you have had UTIs before. Take showers instead of baths.
- Don't wear tight-fitting under garments, jeans and/ or slacks.
- If you use a diaphragm, clean it after each use.

Urinary Tract Infections, continued

☐ Have your doctor check your diaphragm periodically to make sure it still fits properly. The size may need to be changed if you gain or lose weight or if you have a baby. Replace your diaphragm according to your doctor's advice.

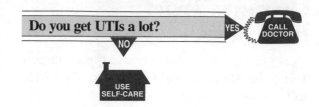

Questions to Ask

Do you have these symptoms?
- **Fever and shaking chills**
- **Pain in one or both sides of your lower back**
- **Vomiting and nausea**

YES → SEEK EMERGENCY CARE

NO

Do you have these problems?
- **Burning or stinging feeling when you pass urine**
- **Passing urine a lot more often than usual**
- **Bloody or cloudy urine**
- **Pain in your abdomen or over your bladder**
- **Sick to your stomach or feeling like you're going to throw up**

YES → SEE DOCTOR

NO

Do you have any of these problems?
- **You feel like you have to go to the bathroom very badly or do you feel like your bladder is still full after you go to the bathroom?**
- **Your urine smell bad?**
- **It hurts to have sex?**

YES → SEE DOCTOR

NO

Have you had symptoms for more than 3 days, without getting better? Did medication the doctor prescribed give you side effects such as a skin rash or make you sick?

YES → CALL DOCTOR

NO

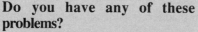

flowchart continued in next column

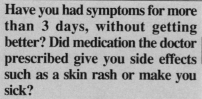

Self-Care Tips

☐ Avoid alcohol, spicy foods, and coffee.

☐ Drink at least 8 glasses of water a day. Cranberry juice is good, too. Liquids help wash out the infection.

☐ Get plenty of rest.

☐ Check for fever twice a day. Take your temperature in the morning and then in the afternoon or evening.

☐ Take aspirin, acetaminophen, ibuprofen, or naproxen sodium. *[Note: Do not give aspirin or any medication containing salicylates to anyone 19 years of age or younger, unless directed by a physician, due to its association with Reye's Syndrome, a potentially fatal condition.]*

☐ Go to the bathroom as soon as you feel the need. Empty your bladder completely, every time you pass urine.
- If you have a condition that keeps you from doing this, such as that which occurs in some persons with multiple sclerosis, ask your doctor about using intermittent self-catheters.

☐ Empty your bladder after sex.

[Note: See your doctor if you don't feel better in 3 days.]

chapter 16

YOUR MENTAL HEALTH

Depression

Life changes, such as the birth of a baby, divorce, death of a loved one, or loss of a job can and do leave people feeling depressed. So can worrying about financial problems or illness. And sometimes you may feel empty and depressed for no apparent reason. Some depression is normal and is a part of almost every person's life. Depression can, however, be a side effect of certain medicines, illnesses, alcoholism, or be a disease in and of itself. Even the lack of natural, unfiltered sunlight between late fall and spring can lead to a type of depression in some sensitive people. This is called Seasonal Affective Disorder (SAD). Depression as a medical disorder affects your thoughts, feelings, physical health and behaviors.

Whatever the cause, depression can be treated. Treatment includes medicines, psychotherapy, and other therapies that are specific to the cause of the depression, such as exposure to bright lights (similar to sunlight) for depression that results from SAD.

Symptoms of depression include:
- ▭ Persistent feelings of sadness or emptiness.
- ▭ Feelings of helplessness, hopelessness, guilt, and worthlessness.
- ▭ Loss of interest in pleasurable activities, including sex.
- ▭ Sleep disturbances.
- ▭ Fatigue.
- ▭ Loss of energy or enthusiasm.
- ▭ Difficulty in concentrating or making decisions.
- ▭ Ongoing physical symptoms, such as headaches or digestive disorders, that don't respond to treatment.
- ▭ Crying, tearfulness.
- ▭ Poor appetite with weight loss, or overeating and weight gain.

Questions To Ask

Have you attempted suicide? Do you have recurrent thoughts of suicide or death? Are you planning ways to commit suicide?

YES → SEEK EMERGENCY CARE

NO ↓

Have you had a loss of interest or pleasure in almost all activities most of the day, nearly every day for at least two weeks? Or, have you been in a depressed mood most of the day, nearly every day and had any of the following, for at least 2 weeks?
- **Feeling slowed down or restless and unable to sit still**
- **Feeling worthless or guilty**
- **Changes in appetite, or weight loss or gain**
- **Thoughts of death or suicide**
- **Problems concentrating, thinking, remembering, or making decisions**
- **Trouble sleeping or sleeping too much**
- **Loss of energy or feeling tired all of the time**
- **Headaches**
- **Other aches and pains**
- **Digestive problems**
- **Sexual problems**
- **Feeling pessimistic or hopeless**
- **Being anxious or worried**

YES → SEE DOCTOR

NO ↓

Has depression interfered with daily activities for more than three weeks? Have you withdrawn from normal activities during this time?

YES → CALL DOCTOR

NO ↓

flowchart continued on next page

Depression, continued

Has the depression appeared after taking over-the-counter or prescription medicine? **YES** CALL DOCTOR

NO

Is the depression associated with dark, cloudy weather, or winter months, and does it lift when spring comes? **YES** CALL DOCTOR

NO

USE SELF-CARE

Self-Care Tips

To overcome mild, hard-to-explain depression, try these approaches:

- Substitute a positive thought for every negative thought that pops into your head.
- Associate with congenial people, not negative people. They'll lift your morale.
- To focus your attention away from yourself, do something to help someone else.
- Get some physical exercise every day, even if it's just taking the dog for a walk. If you can do something more exhilarating, like biking, playing tennis, or chopping firewood, that's even better.
- Do something different. Walk or drive to someplace new, or try a new restaurant.
- Challenge yourself with a new project. It doesn't have to be difficult, but it should be enjoyable. Do something that you enjoy and allows you to express yourself. Examples are writing, painting, etc.
- Do something that will make you relax. Listen to soft music, read a good book, take a warm bath or shower, do relaxation exercises.
- Talk to a friend, relative or co-worker or anyone who will allow you to vent the tensions and frustrations that you are experiencing.
- Avoid drugs and alcohol. Drinking too much alcohol and the use of drugs can cause or worsen depression.

Stress

Stress is the way our bodies react both physically and emotionally to any change in the status quo - good, bad, real or even imagined. Some physical symptoms created by stress include an increased heart rate, rapid breathing, tense muscles, and increased blood pressure. Emotional reactions include irritability, anger, losing one's temper, yelling, lack of concentration, being jumpy, etc. When left unchecked, stress can lead to a variety of health problems including insomnia, ulcers, back pain, colitis, high blood pressure, heart disease, and a lowering of the body's immune system. In fact, the American Academy of Family Physicians states that approximately two thirds of all visits to the family doctor are for stress related disorders.

Questions to Ask

Are you so distressed that you have recurrent thoughts of suicide or death? Do you have impulses or plans to commit violence? **YES** SEEK EMERGENCY CARE

NO

Are you experiencing frequent anxiety, nervousness, crying spells, and confusion about how to handle your problems? **YES** SEE DOCTOR

NO

Are you abusing alcohol, drugs (illegal or prescription) to deal with stress? **YES** SEE DOCTOR

NO

flowchart continued on next page

Stress, continued

Have you been a part of a traumatic event in the past, such as armed combat, airplane crash, rape or assault, etc. and do you now experience any of the following?

- Flashbacks (reliving the stressful event), painful memories, nightmares
- Feeling easily startled and/or irritable
- Feeling "emotionally numb" and detached from others and the outside world
- Having a hard time falling asleep and/or staying asleep
- Anxiety and/or depression

YES 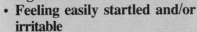 SEE DOCTOR

NO

Do you find yourself withdrawing from friends, relatives and co-workers and/or blowing up at them at the slightest provocation?

YES CALL DOCTOR

NO

Do you suffer from a medical illness that you are unable to cope with? Is this leading you to neglect proper treatment?

YES CALL DOCTOR

NO

 USE SELF-CARE

Self-Care Tips

Being able to manage stress is important in living a healthy, happy, and productive life. Listed below are techniques and strategies to effectively deal with stress:

- Maintain a regular program of healthy eating, good health habits, and adequate sleep.
- Exercise regularly. This promotes physical fitness as well as emotional well being.
- Balance work and play. All work and no play can make you pretty uptight. Plan some time for hobbies and recreation. These activities relax your mind and are a good respite from life's worries.
- Help others. We concentrate on ourselves when we're distressed. Sometimes helping others is the perfect remedy for whatever is troubling us.

- Take a shower or bath with warm water. This will soothe and calm your nerves and relax your muscles.
- Have a good cry. Tears of sadness, joy, or grief can help cleanse the body of substances that accumulate under stress and also release a natural pain relieving substance from the brain.
- Laugh a lot. When events seem too overwhelming, keep a sense of humor. Laughter makes our muscles go limp and releases tension.
- It's difficult to feel stress in the middle of a belly laugh. Learn to laugh as a relaxation technique.
- Learn acceptance. Sometimes a difficult problem is out of your control. When this happens, accept it until changes can be made. This is better than worrying and getting nowhere.
- Talk out troubles. It sometimes helps to talk with a friend, relative or clergyman. Another person can help you see a problem from a different point of view.
- Escape for a little while. When you feel you are getting nowhere with a problem, a temporary diversion can help. Going to a movie, reading a book, visiting a museum or taking a drive can help you get out of a rut. Temporarily leaving a difficult situation can help develop new attitudes.
- Reward yourself. Starting today, reward yourself with little things that make you feel good. Treat yourself to a bubble bath, buy the hardcover edition of a book, call an old friend long distance, buy a flower, picnic in the park during lunchtime, try a new perfume or cologne, or give yourself some "me" time.
- Do a relaxation exercise daily. Good ones include visualization (imagining a soothing, restful scene), deep muscle relaxation (tensing and relaxing muscle fibers), meditation, and deep breathing.
- Budget your time. Make a "to-do list". Prioritize your daily tasks. Avoid committing yourself to doing too much.
- Develop and maintain a positive attitude. View changes as positive challenges, opportunities or blessings.
- Rehearse for stressful events. Imagine yourself feeling calm and confident in an anticipated stressful situation. You will be able to relax more easily when the situation arises.
- Modify your environment to get rid of or manage your exposure to things that cause stress.

chapter 17

CHILDREN'S HEALTH

Bed-wetting

Wetting the bed is not only uncomfortable, it is embarrassing, especially for a child older than 3 years. And that's not all. Afraid of waking up in a soaked bed, children who wet their beds may avoid going to pajama parties, friends' houses or summer camp.

Three out of four toddlers stay dry all night by age 3-1/2. By age 5 years, one in five still wets the bed and at age 6, the numbers drop to one in ten. Just about all bed-wetting stops by the time children reach puberty. Boys are more likely to wet their beds than girls. Bed-wetting may start again during stressful times.

No one really knows what causes enuresis, the medical term for bed-wetting. From the 1930s through the 1960s, it was commonly believed that children who wet their beds had psychological problems. Today, it is suspected that bed-wetting may be caused by slow development of the nerves that control the bladder.

Even a small bladder unable to hold the urine produced during the night can result in bed-wetting. Bed-wetting can be a symptom of an serious illness such as diabetes or a urinary tract infection, especially if it starts in a child who has previously been dry through the night.

Questions to Ask

Does your child drink an excessive amount of fluids, urinate more than usual during the day and night and/or show other signs such as fatigue, increased appetite and weight gain and itching around the genitals? YES

NO

flowchart continued in next column

Does your child have a fever, abdominal pain or burning when urinating? YES

NO

Is your child older than 6 years and never been dry at night or has he or she been dry at night for an extended time and is now wetting again? YES

NO

USE SELF-CARE

Self-Care Tips

Your patience and love will go a long way to help a child who wets the bed. Children have no control over this condition; they don't wet the bed on purpose. Making them feel guilty, getting angry or acting disgusted will only delay solving this problem. Try to be understanding and supportive.

Psychologists recommend that you simply wait it out. Don't praise them for a dry bed nor punish them when it's wet. To help make life easier for your child and yourself, consider the following:

- Have your child change the bed as well as his or her bed clothes during the night, if he or she is able to do so. Or, keep a flannel-covered rubber sheet nearby so your child can put it over the wet sheets.
- Set an alarm clock two to three hours after your child falls asleep so he or she can be awakened to go to the bathroom.
- Make sure your child urinates before getting into bed.

Bed-wetting, continued

- ☐ Encourage your child to follow instructions, if any, that the doctor suggests such as bladder-stretching or stream-interruption exercises, or behavior modification devices.
- ☐ Obtain a bed-wetting alarm. (This is best suited for children 5 years and older). Modern enuresis alarms have moisture sensors that attach directly on the underwear. At the first drop of liquid, a buzzer sounds, waking up the child. Eventually, kids learn to wake up whenever they feel the urge to urinate. Newer models of these alarms can help prevent wet beds about 85 to 90 percent of the time.

Bed wetting alarms and information can be obtained from:

- ☐ Nite Train'r Alarm: Koregon Enterprises, 9735 S.W. Sunshine Court, Beaverton, OR 97005, or call 800-544 4240.
- ☐ Nytone Alarm: Nytone Medical Products, 2424 South 900 West, Salt Lake City, UT 84119, or call 801-973-4090.
- ☐ Wet-Stop Alarm: Palco Laboratories, 8030 Soquel Ave., Santa Cruz, CA 95062, or call 800-346-4488.

Also, check with local home medical supply companies and local pharmacies that carry or can provide home medical equipment.

Chicken Pox

Chicken pox is a very contagious disease caused by a virus (Varicella/herpes zoster). It is spread from child to child, and sometimes to adults, by sneezing, coughing, contaminated clothing and direct contact with open blisters. Children exposed to the virus get chicken pox 7-21 days later.

Most of the time there are no symptoms before the rash appears. Some children, though, may be tired, have a fever and complain of a stomach ache a day or two before a flat, red rash appears. The rash generally begins on the scalp, face and back, but can spread to any body surface. It is rarely seen, though, on the palms of hands or soles of feet. Sores smaller than a pencil eraser, that are sometimes encrusted, can also be found in the mouth, on the eyelids and in the genital area.

Within hours, these flat, red spots turn into tiny clear blisters that itch a lot. As your child scratches the blisters, serum spills out, dries and forms hard crusts that loosen and drop off about two weeks later. Since the rash continues to break out for the first two to six days, new red spots are often seen alongside old dried scabs. Some children have very few spots while others are covered.

Most children recover from chicken pox uneventfully in less than two weeks. Complications are rare, although chicken pox can occasionally lead to encephalitis (an inflammation of the brain), meningitis or pneumonia. Children who have cancer and those who take medications that affect the immune system are at a higher risk of complications from chicken pox. The biggest problem parents face with chicken pox, though, is infected blisters.

There is prescription medication available that can decrease the length and severity of chicken pox. It is not recommended for routine cases. Also, it is only effective if started within 24 hours of the onset of the infection. It does not interfere with the child's developing immunity to chicken pox. Ask your doctor for more information.

One attack of chicken pox usually gives your child lifelong immunity. Children rarely have a second round of chicken pox, but if it does occur, the attacks are usually very mild.

Prevention

A vaccine has been developed for chicken pox. It is called Varicella Zoster Virus Vaccine. Ask your child's health care provider about it. (See "Immunizations" on page 18.)

Chicken Pox, continued

Questions to Ask

Does your child have a severe headache, stiff neck, convulsions, abnormal behavior and/or continuous vomiting? YES

NO

Is your child hard to wake, confused or having trouble breathing? YES

NO

Does your child have cancer, or is your child taking medications that affect the immune system and have a fever higher than 102°F? YES

NO

Does your child have cancer, or is your child taking medications that affect the immune system but not have a fever higher than 102°F? YES

NO

Does your child have a fever higher than 103°F or had a fever higher than 102°F for more than two days? YES

NO

Does your child have any scabs that are red, oozing pus, or bleeding or has he or she developed a red rash with tiny pink dots? YES

NO

Self-Care Tips

The goals are to make your child comfortable and to reduce and relieve the itching so your child does not scratch off the scabs, which could start a secondary infection and/or leave scars.

- Encourage your child not to scratch the scabs. Keep him or her busy with other activities.

- Give your child a cool bath without soap every 3-4 hours for the first couple of days (15-20 minutes at a time). Add one-half cup of baking soda or colloidal oatmeal bath packet such as Aveeno to the bath water. Pat, do not rub, your child dry.

- Dip a washcloth in cool water and place it on the itchy areas.

- Apply calamine (not caladryl) lotion for temporary relief.

- Trim your child's fingernails to prevent infection caused by opened blisters. Scratching off the crusty scabs may leave permanent scars.

- Cover the hands of infants with cotton socks if they are scratching their sores.

- Wash your child's hands three times a day with an antibacterial soap such as Safeguard or Dial to avoid infecting the open blisters.

- Keep your child cool and calm. Heat and sweating makes the itching worse. Also, keep your child out of the sun. Extra chicken pox will occur on parts of the skin exposed to the sun.

- Give your child Benadryl, an over-the counter antihistamine, if the itching is severe or stops your child from sleeping. (See label for proper dosage).

- Give your child acetaminophen (children's versions of the following: Tylenol, Tempra, Liquiprin, Datril, Anacin 3 or Panadol) for the fever. *[Note: Do not give aspirin or any medication containing salicylates to anyone 19 years of age or younger, unless directed by a physician, due to its association with Reye's Syndrome, a potentially fatal condition.]*

- Give your child soft foods and cold fluids if he or she has sores in the mouth. Do not offer salty foods or citrus fruits that may irritate the sores.

- Have your child gargle with salt water (1/4 teaspoon to 4 ounces of water) to help ease itching in the mouth, if necessary.

- Reassure your child that the "bumps" are not serious and will go away in a week or so.

Colic

Colic is one of the most frustrating conditions parents deal with. Your baby cries for hours on end for no apparent reason, tucking those tiny knees close to the stomach as if in severe pain. Typically, the attacks start in the evening when you're most tired and your patience is thin.

Nothing seems to stop the screaming of a colicky infant - not even feeding, changing the diaper or cuddling. Take comfort, though. Colic is rarely dangerous and doesn't last a long time. It usually begins after an infant is two weeks old, peaks at about three months of age and most often ends by the fourth month.

The cause of colic is a mystery. Some pediatricians think it is due to an underdeveloped digestive tract. Others blame food allergies, abdominal gas, not enough sleep or over sensitivity to a busy and noisy home. Still others think it is a combination of these factors. An attack of colic may end with the passage of gas or stool.

Once in a while, colic may be an early sign of a serious medical problem. For example, in the medical condition call intussusception, the bowel becomes obstructed. A doctor can examine your baby and run laboratory tests to check for this and other medical conditions.

Prevention

- ▭ Have your infant sit rather than lie down at feeding time to avoid swallowing air.
- ▭ If breast feeding, watch your intake of caffeine drinks like colas, coffee, cocoa and tea.
- ▭ Stop eating milk products on a one-week trial basis. One study showed that when the mother stopped eating dairy foods, her baby's colic often disappeared. (If you do this, check with your doctor about taking calcium supplements).
- ▭ Do not overheat the milk or formula.
- ▭ Make sure the bottle's nipple holes are not too small. Tiny holes cause babies to swallow air as they suck on the nipples.
- ▭ Try a different type of formula, i.e., a soy-based one instead of one made with cow's milk.
- ▭ Make mealtime a quiet, calm time.
- ▭ Feed more frequently. Burp your baby more often.

Questions to Ask

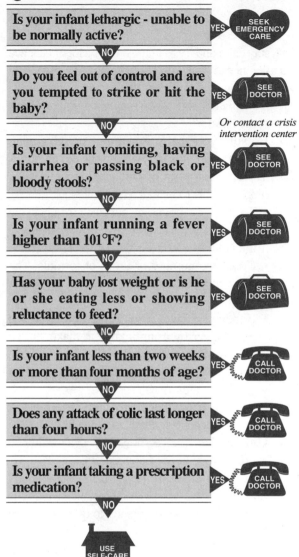

Is your infant lethargic - unable to be normally active? YES → SEEK EMERGENCY CARE

NO

Do you feel out of control and are you tempted to strike or hit the baby? YES → SEE DOCTOR

Or contact a crisis intervention center

NO

Is your infant vomiting, having diarrhea or passing black or bloody stools? YES → SEE DOCTOR

NO

Is your infant running a fever higher than 101°F? YES → SEE DOCTOR

NO

Has your baby lost weight or is he or she eating less or showing reluctance to feed? YES → SEE DOCTOR

NO

Is your infant less than two weeks or more than four months of age? YES → CALL DOCTOR

NO

Does any attack of colic last longer than four hours? YES → CALL DOCTOR

NO

Is your infant taking a prescription medication? YES → CALL DOCTOR

NO

USE SELF-CARE

See Self-Care Tips on next page

Colic, continued

Self-Care Tips

First, stay calm and try to relax. It takes a lot of patience and tolerance to deal with a screaming baby, especially when nothing seems wrong. While none of these self-care tips will cure colic, they may bring you and your baby some relief.

- ☐ Be sure your baby is getting enough to eat. Hunger, not colic, may be causing the crying.
- ☐ Try different types of purchased nipples. If the nipple hole is too small, enlarge it.
  - To check the hole size, put cold formula in the bottle and turn it upside down. Shake or squeeze the bottle.
  - Count the number of drops of formula. The right sized hole delivers about one drop per second.
  - If there are fewer drops per second, make the hole bigger by using a knife to make a cross cut over the existing hole.
- ☐ Hold your child up for feeding and for a short while afterwards.
- ☐ Burp your baby after each ounce of formula or every few minutes when breast feeding.
- ☐ Use a pacifier. (Never, however, put a pacifier on a string around your baby's neck).
- ☐ Wrap your infant in a cozy blanket and gently rock him or her, or use an automatic swing. The back and forth motion tends to quiet a wailing baby.
- ☐ Try what is called the "colic carry". Carefully place your baby face down, with his/her face on your open hand and legs straddling your inner elbow. Support your baby by holding his/her back with your other hand and walk around the house for a while.
- ☐ Vacuum while carrying your infant in a "baby carrier" worn on your chest. Apparently, the noise of a running vacuum soothes a colicky baby.
- ☐ Play soothing music. This may benefit you as well as the baby.
- ☐ Take your baby for a ride outdoors in the stroller or in the car.
- ☐ Run the dryer or dishwasher. Put your baby in an infant seat and lean it against the side of the dryer or on the counter close to the dishwasher. (Stay with your baby and make sure the baby will not be harmed by the heat or steam given off by these appliances). The vibration may put your child to sleep.
- ☐ Do not give the baby liquid antacids (such as Maalox) or simethicone drops. These have not been shown to be helpful.
- ☐ Let your baby cry himself or herself to sleep if none of the above suggestions work. (Don't let your baby cry, however, for more than four hours).
- ☐ If you're stressed, let someone else take over the care of your child for awhile. Get some rest.

Croup

What could be more frightening than to awaken during the night to the sound of your child gasping for air and "barking like a seal". Yet these are the classical signs of croup, a respiratory infection that typically affects children between the ages of 3 months and 3 years. While it may sound frightening, croup is rarely cause for concern. Croup usually lasts from 3 to 7 days. Generally, it worsens at night and tends to improve during the day. Sometimes steroid medication that is prescribed early in the illness helps to ease the severity of the symptoms.

A virus is the most common cause of croup. Infected by a virus, cells in the voice box and windpipe react by secreting mucous that narrow these air passages. The secretions dry and thicken, making it even more difficult for your child to breathe. Dissolving the dried secretions with steam is often all that is needed to relieve your child's discomfort. Children usually outgrow croup as they get older and the windpipe becomes wider.

Croup, continued

Sometimes croup is confused with another condition called epiglottitis (an inflammation of the structure behind the root of the tongue). Typically seen in children older than three years, epiglottitis is often more serious than croup because it can completely block the airway and cause meningitis (an inflammation of the lining of the brain and spinal cord), or respiratory arrest. Children with epiglottitis tend to drool, tilt their heads forward, have a fever and jut their jaw out as they try to breathe.

Sometimes what sounds like croup may instead indicate that your child has inhaled a foreign object. If the object blocks the windpipe, your child will have trouble breathing and will need immediate emergency care.

Prevention

- Run a humidifier near your child's bed for several nights after the first attack. Use a cool mist vaporizer if your child has a fever because warm moist air can raise body temperature. Clean the vaporizer after each use.
- Purchase a humidifier for your furnace if croup is a recurring problem. Change the filter often.

Questions to Ask

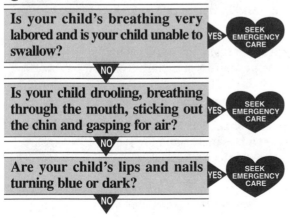

flowchart continued in next column

If you child is making a sound like a barking seal and finding it hard to breathe have you used steam for more than 15 minutes and taken your child outside in the cold night air for 15 minutes **without** getting relief for your child's symptoms? **YES** SEEK EMERGENCY CARE

NO

Is your child making a sound like a barking seal? **YES** SEE DOCTOR

NO

USE SELF-CARE

Self-Care Tips

- Try not to panic. While wheezing and barking sounds are frightening, remaining calm will lessen your child's fear and anxiety.
  - Hold your child to comfort him or her. Helping your child to relax may help stop the windpipe from constricting and make breathing easier.
- Use a hot bath or shower to help relieve the congestion:
  - Take your child to the bathroom and close the door.
  - Turn on the hot water in the sink and shower to fill the room with steam.
  - Do not put your child in the shower. Instead, sit your child on the toilet or a chair, but not on the floor. Try reading a book to your child to pass the time and ease any fears.
  - Open the window to let in cool air. This helps to create more steam.
  - Allow a good 15 minutes for the steam to ease the symptoms. If the symptoms continue, carry your child out-of-doors to breathe the cold night air. If this doesn't ease the breathing difficulties, seek emergency care.
- Use a vaporizer in your child's room. Cold-mist vaporizers are preferred because they give off cool air and avoid the risk of scalding with hot water.

Self-Care Tips continued on next page

Croup, continued

- ☐ Clean the vaporizer after each use.
  - Make a "croup tent" by placing the vaporizer under the crib or bed. Drape a blanket over the crib near the child's head, or over an umbrella if your child now sleeps in a bed, to trap the steam. Never leave your child alone while he or she is in a croup tent. Stay awake to monitor your child.
- ☐ Crying is a good sign. It means that your child's symptoms are subsiding. A crying child is able to breathe.

Lice

Head lice are tiny parasites about the size of a sesame seed. These flat, wingless "bugs" survive by sucking human blood. Louse bites cause an intense itching and red spots on the skin that look like mosquito bites. The adult lice are rarely seen. Instead, you see what are called "nits", clusters of lice eggs deposited on hair strands that are often mistaken for dandruff.

Lice spread quickly from person to person by direct contact with someone who has them. No matter how well-groomed and clean your child is, he or she can get them in school, from toilet seats or from anyone who already has them. Female lice lay about six eggs a day. The eggs hatch in eight to ten days, after which they soon begin their annoying biting.

There are three types of lice: Head lice, pubic lice and body lice. All are very attracted to body-heat. Head lice is the most common type, especially among children in day-care centers, camps and schools. Pubic lice, found on the pubic hair, is called the "crabs", because the lice look like crabs. Body lice live in the seams of dirty clothes and bedding.

Prevention

To prevent head lice, children should be told:
- ☐ Not to share hats, brushes or combs.
- ☐ Not to lie on a pillow shared with another child.
- ☐ To shampoo their hair and to bathe frequently.

You should:
- ☐ Change bed linens often and wash them in hot water and dry them in a dryer, especially during an epidemic of lice at school.
- ☐ Vacuum furniture, mattresses, rugs, stuffed animals and car seats if anyone in your family is infected with lice. Do not use insecticidal sprays for lice.
- ☐ Immediately notify anyone who may have been in close contact with your child to help prevent infecting others with lice. Be sure to contact:
  - Your child's school.
  - Your child care provider.
  - Parents of your child's friends.
  - Neighbors.
- ☐ Wash combs and brushes. Then soak them in hot, not boiling, water for 10 minutes.
- ☐ Check your children for head lice and nits at least once a week. Check more often if your child is scratching his or her head. Look for nits around the nape of the neck and behind the ears. Use two round toothpicks to spread hairs apart to look for nits.

Questions to Ask

Are there open wounds on your child's scalp caused by scratching? YES

NO

Have you found lice or nits in your child's eyebrows or eyelashes or on the hair shaft or skin? YES

NO

Does your child's scalp itch, do you see red bite marks and are lymph glands in the neck swollen? YES

NO

flowchart continued on next page

Lice, continued

If your child has lice, does he or she have allergies or other health problems, or is your child under 2 years of age? **YES** → **CALL DOCTOR**

NO ↓

USE SELF-CARE

Self-Care Tips

Only insecticidal shampoos, lotions and creams kill lice. You can buy these products over-the-counter at your drug store. Your doctor can also prescribe medication to treat lice and kill the nits. All lice-killing products are pesticides, so must be used with caution and only as directed.

Everyone in your household should be checked for lice and nits. However, only treat those who are infested. Lice killing products are not to be used to prevent infestation.

When using an insecticidal shampoo:
- ▭ Follow the directions exactly as given, and:
  - Remove your child's shirt.
  - Give your child a towel to cover his or her eyes. Do not use the shampoo around your child's eyes.
  - Lean your child over the sink as you apply the shampoo. Do not put your child in the shower or bathtub; the shampoo should only be applied to the head and neck.
- ▭ Don't use too much shampoo or you'll make your child's scalp too dry.
- ▭ If you have open sores on your hands, wear gloves or have someone else shampoo your child's hair.

To remove the nits:
- ▭ Shine a flashlight into the scalp, or other infected body part. Nits may be gray and hard to see. If your child has blonde hair, check your child's scalp carefully because the nits will be harder to find.

- ▭ Begin in one part of the scalp and move row by row, even strand by strand, when necessary.
- ▭ Remove nits from the hair strands with tweezers, safety manicure scissors, a nit-comb (available at the drug store), or your fingernails. Some products come with a fine-toothed comb you can use to dislodge the nits.
  - Before using the comb, dip it in hot vinegar. This will help loosen the nits.
  - Comb the hair from the scalp toward the ends. After each pass, check the comb for nits.
  - Or, using hair clips to hold the hair, separate it into 4 to 5 sections. Starting in one section, lift about an inch of hair upward and outward. Place the comb on the scalp and comb the hair from the scalp to its tip. Repeat for each section of hair.
  - Soak all combs, brushes and barrettes for several hours in the insecticidal shampoo or for 10 minutes in hot water.

Check for nits every day for about 10 days.
If necessary, shampoo again a week later to kill any newly hatched nits. It is not necessary to remove nits after treatment is completed, except for cosmetic purposes.

You should also:
- ▭ Immediately wash bedding and clothing in water hotter than 125°F. Heat kills the lice and destroys the nits. If an item cannot be washed, put it in an airtight plastic bag and seal. Do not open it for at least two weeks. Deprived of blood, the lice will die.
- ▭ Dry clean clothing and hats that cannot be washed.
- ▭ Vacuum all mattresses, pillows, rugs and upholstered furniture, especially in areas where children play. Using the long, narrow attachment, suck lice or nits out of car seats, toys, stuffed animals and other small areas. Dispose of the vacuum cleaner bags.

chapter 18
WOMEN'S HEALTH

Breast Cancer & Breast Self-Exam

Breast cancer is the most common form of cancer among women, accounting for 30% of cancers women get. Each year, there are approximately 185,000 new cases of breast cancer and 45,000 deaths from it. Only lung cancer causes more cancer deaths among women. The chance of breast cancer increases dramatically with age. The National Cancer Institute (NCI) has given the following statistics for a woman's chances of developing breast cancer:

By Age	Chances
25	1 in 19,608
30	1 in 2,525
35	1 in 622
40	1 in 217
45	1 in 93
50	1 in 50
55	1 in 33
60	1 in 24
65	1 in 17
70	1 in 14
75	1 in 11
80	1 in 10
85	1 in 9
Lifetime	1 in 8

Men can also develop breast cancer, but it is very unusual. About 300 men die each year from the disease.

Breast cancer results from malignant tumors which invade and destroy normal tissue. When these tumors break away and spread to other parts of the body, it is called metastasis. Breast cancers can spread to the lymph nodes, lungs, liver, bone and brain.

The risk of breast cancer increases above the normal risk with these factors:

- Having had breast cancer increases the risk for cancer in the remaining breast tissue.
- Never giving birth or giving birth after age 30.
- Early onset of menstruation (before age 12).
- Late menopause (after age 55).
- Family history of breast cancer - mother, daughter or sister has had the disease. The risk increases even more if the relative's cancer came prior to menopause or if affected both breasts.
- Exposure to radiation.
- Diet high in fat.
- Being overweight (for older women only).

Detection

Early screening for breast cancer includes:

- Mammograms. Make sure you have mammograms at facilities that are accredited by the American College of Radiology (ACR). Call The National Cancer Institute Hotline at 1-800-4-CANCER to find ones in your area.
- Clinical breast exams.
- Breast self-exams.

If a lump or other problem is found, the doctor can do further exams and tests to check for cancer.

Treatment

There are a variety of treatments for breast cancer. The main treatment is surgery. The removal of the cancerous area is most often recommended along with taking a sample of the lymph nodes in the armpit to see if the cancer has spread there.

Breast Cancer &
Breast Self-Exam, continued

Other treatments are radiation therapy, chemotherapy and hormonal therapy. It is important to find out the type of cancer cell that is involved. If the cancer is a type which spreads quickly, a more extensive surgical treatment may be chosen.

Types of Surgical Procedures:

Lumpectomy - the lump and a border of surrounding tissue are removed.

Partial or segmental mastectomy - the tumor and up to one-fourth of the breast tissue are removed.

Simple or total mastectomy - the entire breast is removed.

Modified radial mastectomy - the entire breast, the underarm lymph nodes and the lining covering the chest muscles, but not the muscles themselves, are removed.

Radical mastectomy - the breast, lymph nodes in the armpit and the chest muscles under the breast are removed.

Ask your doctor about the benefits and risks for each surgical option and decide together which option is best for you.

Questions to Ask

Do you see or feel any lumps, thickening or changes of any kind when you examine your breasts? For example, is there dimpling, puckering, retraction of the skin or change in the shape or contour of the breast? YES

NO

Do you have breast pain or a constant tenderness that lasts throughout the menstrual cycle? YES

NO

Do the nipples become drawn into the chest or are they inverted totally, change shape or become crusty from a discharge? YES

NO

flowchart continued on next page

If you normally have lumpy breasts (already diagnosed as being benign by your doctor), do you notice any new lumps or have any lumps changed in size or are you concerned about having "benign" lumps? YES

NO

Is there any non-milky discharge when you squeeze the nipple of either breast or both breasts? YES

NO

Do you have a family history of breast cancer which leads you to be concerned even if you don't notice any problems when you examine your breasts? YES

NO

Have you had recent trauma which results in a breast lump being formed? YES

NO

*Continue to Perform
Breast Self-Examination Monthly and
Use Self-care and Prevention Tips
on Page 138*

How to Examine Your Breasts

It is normal to have some lumpiness or thickening in the breasts. By examining your breasts once each month, you will learn what is normal for you and notice when any changes do occur. Some women find that doing a daily or weekly self-exam works better for them. They learn their breasts at all phases of their menstrual cycle. The more you can examine your breasts, the better you can learn what is normal for you. Your "job" isn't just to find lumps, but to notice if there are any changes.

Breast Cancer & Breast Self-Exam, continued

In the shower - With your fingers flat, gently move the

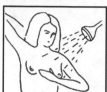

pads of your fingertips over every part of each breast. Use your right hand to examine the left breast and your left hand to examine the right breast. Check for any thickening, hard lump, or knot.

In front of a mirror - Holding your arms at your sides,

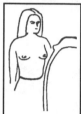

look at your breasts. Raise your arms overhead. Look for any changes in the shape of each breast, swelling, dimpling, or changes in the nipples.

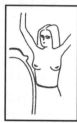

Lying down - To examine your right breast, put a

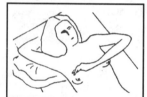

pillow under your right shoulder. Place your right hand behind your head. Then, using the fingers of your left hand held flat, press gently in small circular motions around an imaginary clock face. Begin at the outermost top of your right breast for 12 o'clock, then move to 10 o'clock, etc. until you get back to 12 o'clock. Each breast will have a normal ridge of firm tissue. Then

move in one inch toward the nipple, including the nipple. Keep circling to examine every part of your breast including the nipple. Repeat the procedure on the left breast with a pillow under the left shoulder and your left hand behind your head. Finally, squeeze the nipple of each breast gently between the thumb and index finger. Any clear or bloody discharge should be reported to your physician immediately.

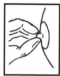

Self-Care and Prevention Tips

☐ Follow a low fat diet. Focus on fresh fruits and vegetables, whole grains, etc.

☐ Eat vegetables that contain a substance called sulforaphane, which may help protect against breast cancer. Examples: broccoli, cabbage, cauliflower, and brussels sprouts.

☐ Avoid unnecessary X-rays. Wear a lead apron when you get dental X-rays and other X-rays not of the chest.

☐ Breast-feed your babies. This may reduce your risk for breast cancer, especially before menopause.

☐ Limit alcohol.

Menopause

Menopause is when a woman's menstrual periods stop altogether. It signals the end of fertility. A woman is said to have gone through menopause when her menstrual periods have stopped for an entire year. "The change" as menopause is often called, generally occurs between the ages of 45 and 55. It can, though, occur as early as 35 or as late as 65 years of age. It can also result from the surgical removal of both ovaries. The physical and emotional signs and symptoms that go with "the change" usually span 1-2 years or more (peri-menopause). They vary from woman to woman. The changes themselves are a result of a number of factors. These include hormone changes, such as estrogen decline, the aging process itself, and stress.

Physical signs and symptoms associates with menopause are:

☐ Hot flashes - sudden waves of heat that can start in the waist or chest and work their way to the neck and face and sometimes the rest of the body. They are more common in the evening and during hot weather. They can hit as often as every 90 minutes. Each one can last from 15 seconds to 30 minutes - 5 minutes is average. Seventy-five to eighty percent of women going through menopause experience hot flashes, some more bothered by them than others. Sometimes heart palpitations accompany hot flashes.

Menopause, continued

- ☐ Irregular periods - this varies and can include:
  - Periods that get shorter and lighter for two or more years.
  - Periods that stop for a few months and then start up again and are more widely spaced.
  - Periods that bring heavy bleeding and/or the passage of many or large blood clots. This can lead to anemia.
- ☐ Vaginal dryness - this results from hormone changes. The vaginal wall also becomes thinner. These problems can make sexual intercourse painful or uncomfortable and can lead to irritation and increased risk for infection.
- ☐ Loss of bladder tone which can result in stress incontinence (leaking urine when you cough, sneeze, laugh or exercise).
- ☐ Headaches, dizziness.
- ☐ Skin and hair changes. Skin is more likely to wrinkle. Growth of facial hair, but thinning of hair in the temple region.
- ☐ Muscles lose some strength and tone.
- ☐ Bones become more brittle, increasing the risk for osteoporosis.
- ☐ Risk for a heart attack increases when estrogen levels drop.

Emotional changes associated with menopause:
- ☐ Irritability.
- ☐ Mood changes.
- ☐ Lack of concentration, difficulty with memory.
- ☐ Tension, anxiety, depression.
- ☐ Insomnia which may result from hot flashes that interrupt sleep.

Treatment for the symptoms of menopause varies from woman to woman. If symptoms cause little or no distress, medical treatment is not needed. Self-Care Tips (see next column) may be all that is required. Hormone replacement therapy (HRT) can reduce many of the symptoms of menopause. It also offers significant protection against osteoporosis and heart disease. The risk for heart attacks, for example, is reduced by 50% with HRT. Each woman should discuss the benefits and risks of HRT with her doctor. (See "Osteoporosis" on page 172 and "Chest Pain" on page 113.)

Medication to treat depression and/or anxiety may be warranted in some women. Also, certain sedative medicines can help with hot flashes.

Questions to Ask

Do you have any of these?
- **Extreme pain during intercourse**
- **Pain or burning when urinating**
- **Thick, white or colored vaginal discharge**
- **Fever and/or chills**

YES SEE DOCTOR

NO ▼

Do you have heavy bleeding with your periods or pass many small clots or large ones which can leave you pale and very tired?

YES CALL DOCTOR

NO ▼

Have you begun menstrual periods again after going without one for six months?

YES CALL DOCTOR

NO ▼

Are hot flashes severe, frequent or persistent enough that they interfere with normal activities?

YES CALL DOCTOR

NO ▼

Do you have risk factors for osteoporosis?
- **Family history of osteoporosis**
- **Small bone frame**
- **Thin**
- **Fair skin (Caucasian or Asian race)**
- **Had surgery to remove ovaries before normal menopause or menopause before 48 years of age**
- **Lack of calcium in diet**
- **Lack of weight-bearing exercise**
- **Alcohol abuse**
- **Hyperthyroidism**
- **Use of steroid medicine**

YES CALL DOCTOR

NO

flowchart continued in next column

If taking hormone replacement therapy (HRT), are you having any of the following?
• Side effects
• Return of menopausal symptoms

YES → CALL DOCTOR

NO ↓

USE SELF-CARE

Self-Care Tips

To reduce the discomfort of hot flashes, try these tactics:

☐ Wear lightweight clothes made of natural fibers.

☐ Limit or avoid beverages that contain caffeine or alcohol.

☐ Avoid rich and spicy foods and heavy meals.

☐ Have cool drinks, especially water, when you feel a hot flash coming on and before and after exercising. Avoid hot drinks.

☐ Keep cool. Open a window. Lower the thermostat when the heat is on. Use air conditioning and/or fans. Carry a small fan with you (hand or battery operated).

☐ Try to relax when you get a hot flash. Getting stressed out over one only makes it worse.

☐ Use relaxation techniques such as meditation, biofeedback or yoga.

☐ Take 400 international units of vitamin E daily, but consult your doctor first.

If you suffer from night sweats, (hot flashes that occur as you sleep):

☐ Wear loose fitting cotton nightwear. Have changes of nightwear ready.

☐ Sleep with only a top sheet, not blankets.

☐ Keep the room cool.

To deal with vaginal dryness and painful intercourse:

☐ Don't use deodorant soaps or scented products in the vaginal area.

☐ Use a water soluble lubricant such as K-Y Jelly, Replens, etc. to facilitate penetration during intercourse. Avoid oils or petroleum-based products. They encourage infection.

☐ Ask your doctor about intravaginal estrogen cream.

☐ Remain sexually active. Having sex often may lessen the chance of having the vagina constrict, help keep natural lubrication and maintain pelvic muscle tone. This includes reaching orgasm with a partner or alone.

☐ Avoid using antihistamines unless truly necessary. They dry mucus membranes in the body.

To deal with emotional symptoms:

☐ Exercise regularly. This will help maintain your body's hormonal balance and preserve bone strength.

☐ Talk to other women who have gone through or are going through menopause. You can help each other cope with emotional symptoms.

☐ Avoid stressful situations as much as possible.

☐ Use relaxation techniques. Examples include: meditation, yoga, listening to soft music and massages.

☐ Eat a healthy diet. Check with your doctor about taking vitamin/mineral supplements.

Menstrual Cramps

Menstrual cramps are also called dysmenorrhea or painful periods. Most women experience them at some time during their life. They can range from very mild to severe. They may also differ from month to month or year to year. The pain felt during menstrual cramps may be accompanied by backache, fatigue, vomiting, diarrhea and headaches. It can be made worse by premenstrual bloating (water retention).

There are two types of dysmenorrhea - primary and secondary. The primary form usually occurs in females who have just begun to menstruate. It may disappear or become less severe after a woman reaches her mid-twenties or gives birth. (Childbirth stretches the uterus.) The cause of menstrual cramps is thought to be related to hormone-like substances called prostaglandins. These are chemicals that occur naturally in the body. Certain prostaglandins cause muscles in the uterus to go into spasms.

Menstrual Cramps, continued

Dysmenorrhea occurs much less often in women who do not ovulate. For this reason, oral contraceptives reduce painful periods in 70-80% of women who take them. When the pill is stopped, women usually get the same level of pain they had before they took it.

Seconcary dysmenorrhea refers to menstrual cramps that are due to other disorders of the reproductive system such as fibroids, endometriosis, ovarian cysts and rarely, cancer. Having an intrauterine device (IUD), especially if you've never been pregnant, can also cause menstrual cramps, except with the Progestasert IUD. It releases a small amount of progesterone into the uterus which helps with cramps and lightens menstrual flow.

Questions to Ask

Have your menstrual periods been especially painful since having an intrauterine contraceptive device (IUD) inserted? YES SEE DOCTOR

NO

Do you have any signs of infection such as fever and foul smelling vaginal discharge or do you have black stools or blood in the stools? YES SEE DOCTOR

NO

For women who are still capable of bearing children: Do you have a heavier than usual blood flow or is your period late by one or more weeks? YES CALL DOCTOR

NO

Is the pain extreme or have you had pain-free periods for years, but are now having severe cramps? YES CALL DOCTOR

NO

Does cramping continue even after your period is over? YES CALL DOCTOR

NO

USE SELF-CARE

Self-Care Tips

To relieve menstrual cramps:

- Take over-the-counter ibuprofen or naproxen sodium around the clock as directed to relieve pain and inhibit the release of prostaglandins. Acetaminophen will help with pain, but not with prostaglandins. Most over-the-counter menstrual discomfort products contain acetaminophen. Read labels. *[Note: Do not give aspirin or any medication containing salcylates to anyone 19 years of age or younger, unless directed by a physician, due to its association with Reye's Syndrome, a potentially fatal condition.]*
- Drink a hot cup of regular tea, chamomile or mint tea.
- Hold a heating pad or hot-water bottle on your abdomen or lower back.
- Take a warm bath.
- Gently massage your abdomen.
- Do mild exercises like stretching, yoga, walking or biking. Exercise may improve blood flow and reduce pelvic pain.
- Whenever possible, lie on your back, supporting your knees with a pillow.
- Unless you have reasons to avoid alcohol, have a glass of wine or other alcoholic beverage. Alcohol slows down uterine contractions.
- Get plenty of rest and avoid stressful situations as your period approaches.
- For birth control, consider using the pill because it blocks the production of prostaglandins or the Progestasert IUD because its use lessens menstrual cramps.

If you still feel pain after using self-care tips, call your doctor.

PMS - Premenstrual Syndrome

Four out of ten menstruating women suffer from PMS (premenstrual syndrome). A syndrome is a group of signs and symptoms that indicate a disorder. There have been as many as 150 symptoms associated with PMS. The most common ones are:

- Irritability.
- Anxiety.

PMS - Premenstrual Syndrome, cont'd

- Depression.
- Headache.
- Bloating.
- Fatigue.
- Feelings of hostility and anger.
- Food cravings, especially for chocolate, sweet and salty foods.

The exact cause or causes for PMS are not known. There are many theories. One points to low levels of the hormone progesterone. Others link it to nutritional or chemical deficiencies. One thing is certain, though, to be classified as PMS, symptoms must occur between ovulation and menstruation; that is, anytime within 2 weeks before the menstrual period and disappear shortly after the period begins.

For some women, symptoms are slight and may last only a few days before menstruation. For others, they can be severe and last the whole two weeks before every period. Also worth noting is that other disorders women experience such as arthritis or clinical depression may be worse during this same premenstrual period. This is known as premenstrual magnification (PMM).

PMS is often confused with depression. An evaluation by your doctor can help with a correct diagnosis. PMS usually stops with menopause:

Treatment for PMS may include:
- Medical management with medicines such as:
  - The prescribed hormone progesterone (suppositories or an oral form).
  - Water pills such as Spironolactone (Aldactone).
  - Antidepressant or antianxiety medicines.
- Dietary measures such as:
  - Eating 5-6 light meals a day instead of 3 large. ones. Not skipping meals.
  - Avoiding sweets.
  - Limiting salt and fat.
  - Avoiding caffeine and alcohol.
  - Vitamin supplements.
  - Adequate intake of calcium and magnesium.
- Lifestyle changes such as: regular exercise which includes 20 minutes of aerobic exercise such as walking or aerobic dance at least 3 times a week.
- Limiting and learning to deal with stress.

Questions to Ask

Are symptoms of PMS such as anxiety, depression and anger that leads to aggression making you feel suicidal? YES → SEEK EMERGENCY CARE

NO ↓

Do PMS symptoms make you feel out of control and unable to live your daily life? YES → SEE DOCTOR

NO ↓

Do you still have PMS symptoms after your period starts? YES → CALL DOCTOR

NO ↓

Have you tried the self-care tips and still don't feel better? YES → CALL DOCTOR

NO ↓

USE SELF-CARE

Self-Care Tips

- Exercise 3 times a week for 20 minutes. Swimming, walking and bicycling all relax your muscles and help you lose water weight.
- Eat 5 - 6 small meals a day instead of 3 large ones. Choose: whole grains, fruits and vegetables; good food sources of calcium such as skim milk, non-fat yogurt, collard greens, kale, calcium-fortified cereals and juices; and sources of magnesium such as spinach, other green, leafy vegetables and whole grain cereals.
- Limit salt, fat and sugar. Doing so may help keep your breasts from getting sore. It may also cut down on your body's estrogen. Estrogen is a hormone that may cause PMS.
- If you need to satisfy a food craving, do so in moderation. For example, if you crave chocolate, have a small chocolate bar or add chocolate syrup to skim milk. If you crave salt, eat a small bag of pretzels.
- Stay away from caffeine, alcohol and cigarettes for 2 weeks before your period is due.

142

PMS - Premenstrual Syndrome, cont'd.

☐ The vitamins and minerals listed here seem to help some women. Ask your doctor if you should take any of them and in what amounts.

- Vitamin E.
- Vitamin B6.
- Calcium.
- Magnesium.
- L-tyrosine, an amino acid.

☐ Take naps if you need to.

☐ Learn to relax. Try deep breathing, meditation, yoga or taking a hot bath.

☐ Try to avoid stress when you have PMS.

Toxic Shock Syndrome

Toxic shock syndrome (TSS) is a potentially fatal disease that is caused by bacteria. It is a form of blood poisoning which results when poisons (toxins) are released by the suspect bacteria. It can result from wounds or infection in the throat, lungs, skin or bone. Most often, though, it affects women of childbearing age, especially women who use super absorbent tampons. These may trap the bacteria and provide a breeding ground for them especially when left in place for along period of time. Also, the super absorbent fibers in some tampons may cause microscopic tears in the vagina that allow the transmission of the bacteria's toxin. Though not common, TSS can also occur in persons following surgery including women who have had a cesarean section. Symptoms come on fast and are often severe. They include:

☐ High sudden fever.

☐ Muscle aches.

☐ Vomiting.

☐ Diarrhea.

☐ Sunburn-like rash, including peeling skin on hands and feet.

☐ Rapid pulse.

☐ Extreme fatigue and weakness.

☐ Sore throat.

☐ Dizziness.

☐ Fainting.

☐ Drop in blood pressure.

Questions to Ask

Are symptoms of toxic shock syndrome present? These could occur during your menstrual period or any other time of month. → YES → SEEK EMERGENCY CARE

NO ↓

USE SELF-CARE

Self-Care Prevention Tips

☐ Never use tampons if you've experienced TSS in the past.

☐ Use sanitary napkins instead of tampons whenever possible.

☐ Alternate tampons with sanitary pads or mini-pads during a menstrual period.

☐ Don't use super absorbent tampons.

☐ Lubricate the tampon applicator with a water-soluble (non-greasy) lubricant like K Y Jelly before insertion.

☐ Change tampons and sanitary pads every 4 to 6 hours or more frequently.

Vaginal Yeast Infections

Yeast infections are the most common type of vaginal infections. Other names for this are Monila, Candida or fungus infection. Vaginal yeast infections result from the overgrowth of Candida albicans which is normally present in harmless amounts in the vagina, the digestive tract and the mouth. Some women rarely have a yeast infection. Others have them regularly. Certain things may trigger them such as:

☐ Hormonal changes that come with pregnancy or even before monthly periods.

Vaginal Yeast Infections, continued

- Taking hormones or birth control pills.
- Taking antibiotics especially "broad spectrum" ones.
- Taking steroid medicines such as prednisone.
- Having elevated blood sugar such as found in uncontrolled diabetes.
- Vaginal intercourse, especially with inadequate lubrication.
- Douching.

Symptoms can range from mild to severe. They include:
- Itching and irritation and redness around the external genitalia.
- A thick, white discharge that looks like cottage cheese and may smell like yeast.
- Burning and/or pain when you urinate or have sex.

Prevention

To help prevent yeast infections:
- Practice good hygiene. Wash regularly to clean the inside folds of the vulva where germs are likely to grow. Dry the vaginal area thoroughly after you shower or bathe.
- Wipe from front to back after using the toilet.
- Wear all-cotton underpants and panty hose with cotton crotches.
- Don't wear slacks and shorts that are tight in the crotch and thighs or other tight fitting clothing such as panty girdles.
- Change underwear and workout clothes right away after exercising.
- Use unscented tampons or sanitary pads and change tampons and sanitary pads frequently.
- Don't use bath oils, bubble baths, feminine hygiene sprays, perfumed or deodorant soaps.
- Don't sit around in a wet bathing suit.
- Shower after you swim in a pool to remove the chlorine from your skin. Dry the vaginal area thoroughly.
- Take antibiotics, especially broad spectrum ones such as Keflex, Ceclor, Bactrim, Septra, amoxicillin, ampicillin, etc. only when necessary to treat bacterial (not viral) infections. These promote the growth of yeast.

- If you tend to get yeast infections whenever you take an antibiotic, ask your doctor to prescribe a vaginal antifungal agent as well or use an over-the-counter one.
- Eat well and include food products such as yogurt that contain live cultures of "lactobacillus acidophilus".
- Get plenty of rest to make it easier for your body to fight infections.

Treatment

Treatment for vaginal yeast infections are:
- Vaginal creams or suppositories that get rid of the Candida overgrowth. These can be over-the-counter ones. Examples are Monistat, Gyne-Lotrimin, etc. or ones prescribed by your doctor such as Terazol or Vagistat, etc. They should be inserted right before you go to bed.
- Oral medicines which include Diflucan (a pill taken once per episode of infection), Sporanox, Nystatin and Nizoral.
- Gentian violet, a purple-colored solution applied to the vaginal area.

It is important, though, to make sure that you have the right problem diagnosed. A burning sensation could be a symptom of a urinary tract infection caused by bacteria which requires an antibiotic. Antibiotics will not help a yeast infection. They make them worse.

Trichomoniasis mimics yeast infections.

You should check with your doctor if:
- This is the first time you have symptoms of a yeast infection.
- You are not sure that your problem is a yeast infection.
- If the infection you treat comes back within two months.
- If the infection does not respond to treatment.

Chronic vaginal infections can be one of the first signs of diabetes, sexually transmitted diseases or HIV/AIDS in women.

Vaginal Yeast Infections, continued

Questions to Ask

Do you have any other symptoms such as vaginal swelling and/or unusual bleeding? Does the discharge have a foul smelling odor? **YES**

NO

Do symptoms of a vaginal yeast infection worsen or continue one week or longer despite using self-care tips or do they come back within 2 months after treatment? **YES**

NO

Self-Care Tips

To get rid of a yeast infection, try the following:

- ▭ Use an over-the-counter vaginal cream medicine or suppositories, such as Monistat, as directed. These used to be available only with a prescription. Women who have had yeast infections whenever they have taken antibiotics in the past should use this during the period of antibiotic treatment.

- ▭ Douche with a mild solution of 1 to 3 tablespoons of vinegar diluted in a quart of warm water. Repeat only once a day until the symptoms subside, but not longer than a week. Too much douching can lead to a flare up of the infection.

- ▭ Limit your intake of sugar and foods that contain sugar since sugar promotes the growth of yeast.

- ▭ Eat yogurt and other food items that contain live cultures of lactobacillus acidophilus several times daily especially when taking an antibiotic. If you can't tolerate yogurt, ask your pharmacist for an over-the-counter product that contains this beneficial bacteria (lactobacillus acidophilus).

chapter 19
MEN'S HEALTH

Enlarged Prostate

The prostate gland is a walnut-shaped organ located below a man's bladder that makes seminal fluid. It actually surrounds a portion of the bladder and the beginning of the urethra, the tube that carries urine away from the bladder.

If they live long enough, most men will eventually get an enlarged prostate gland. Doctors call it benign prostatic hyperplasia (BPH).

An enlarged prostate is usually not cancerous or life threatening. It may cause some problems such as:

- Increased urgency to urinate.
- Frequent urination, especially during the night.
- Delay in onset of urine flow.
- Diminished or slow stream of urine flow.
- Incomplete emptying of the bladder.

These symptoms indicate that the prostate gland has enlarged enough to partially obstruct the flow of urine. Sometimes, BPH causes a urinary tract infection. Over time, a few men might have bladder or kidney problems or both.

Your doctor can diagnose BPH through a number of things. These include:

- A physical exam which includes asking questions about your current symptoms and past medical problems, an examination of your prostate gland, checking your urine for signs of infection and a blood test to see if the prostate has affected your kidneys.
- Tests that measure urine flow, the amount of urine left in your bladder after you urinate and the pressure in your bladder as your urinate.

- A blood test called Prostate-Specific Antigen (PSA) which can help find prostate cancer. Not all doctors agree that being tested for PSA levels lowers a patient's chance of dying from prostate cancer. The PSA test is not always accurate either. You should discuss this test with your doctor.
- Other tests such as X-rays, cystoscopy (the doctor looks directly at the prostate and bladder) and an ultrasound (sound wave pictures of the prostate, kidneys or bladder). Many men do not need these tests. They are costly and are not very helpful for most men with BPH.

Treatment for BPH varies depending on symptoms. Discuss the benefits and possible problems with your doctor for each treatment option. Treatment options include:

- Watchful waiting - getting regular exams to see if your BPH is causing problems or getting worse
- Medications - There are two types:
  - Alpha blockers which help relax muscles in the prostate. Hytrin is one approved for BPH treatment by the Food and Drug Administration (FDA).
  - Finasteride (Proscar) which causes the prostate to shrink

There is no evidence that these medications reduce the rate of BPH complications or the need for future surgery. They can have side effects, too, so you will need to see your doctor for monitoring.

- Balloon dilation - a surgical procedure done in the operating room or doctor's office. A balloon-tipped catheter is inserted into the penis through the urethra and into the bladder. The balloon is inflated to stretch the urethra which aims at allowing urine to flow more easily.

Enlarged Prostate, continued

- [ ] Surgery - There are three types:
  - Transurethral resection of the prostate (TURP). - This type is the most common one done. It relieves symptoms by reducing pressure on the urethra. It is a proven way to treat BPH effectively.
  - Transurethral incision of the prostate (TUIP) - This, too, reduces the prostate's pressure on the urethra making it easier to urinate. TUIP may be used instead of TURP when the prostate is not enlarged as much.
  - Open prostatectomy - This may be used if the prostate is very large. An incision is made in the lower abdomen to remove part of the inside of the prostate.

Prostate surgery can result in problems such as impotence and/or incontinence. It is important to discuss the benefits and the risks of these operations with your doctor. Most men who undergo surgery have no major problems.

Questions to Ask

Do you have one or more of these problems?
- **A feeling that you have to urinate right away or the need to urinate often especially at night**
- **A feeling that you can't empty your bladder completely**
- **A feeling of hesitancy or delay or straining to urinate**
- **A weak or interrupted urinary stream**

 YES → SEE DOCTOR

NO

flowchart continued in next column

Do you have one or more of these symptoms of an infection that may result from BPH?
- **Burning, frequent or painful urination**
- **Pain in the lower back, groin or testicles**
- **Pain in or near the penis**
- **Pain on ejaculation**
- **Discharge from the penis (blood or pus)**
- **Fever and/or chills**

 YES → SEE DOCTOR

NO

USE SELF-CARE

Self-Care Tips

- [ ] Remain sexually active.
- [ ] Take hot baths.
- [ ] Avoid dampness and cold temperatures.
- [ ] Do not let the bladder get too full. Urinate as soon as the urge arises. Relax when you urinate.
- [ ] When you take long care trips, make frequent stops to urinate. Keep a container that you can urinate in when you are riding in a car in the event that you can't get to a bathroom in time.
- [ ] Whenever possible, sit on a hard chair instead of a soft one.
- [ ] Limit coffee, alcohol and foods that are spicy.
- [ ] Drink eight or more glasses of water every day, but don't drink liquids before going to bed.
- [ ] Reduce stress.
- [ ] Don't smoke.
- [ ] Avoid taking over-the-counter antihistamines.

Jock Itch

Symptoms of jock itch are redness, itching and scaliness in the groin and thigh area. Jock itch is usually caused by a fungus infection. It can also result from a bacterial infection or be a reaction to chemicals in clothing, irritating garments or medicines that you take.

Jock itch gets its name because an athletic supporter worn during a workout then stored in a dark, poorly ventilated locker and then work again without being laundered, provides the ideal environment in which the fungi thrive. (Under similar conditions, women's clothing can develop this problem, too.)

Questions to Ask

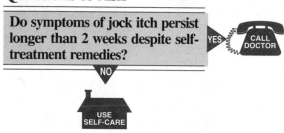

Do symptoms of jock itch persist longer than 2 weeks despite self-treatment remedies?

YES → CALL DOCTOR

NO → USE SELF-CARE

Self-Care Tips

To relieve jock itch and prevent future attacks:

- Don't wear tight, close-fitting clothing. Boxer shorts are recommended for men.
- Change underwear frequently, especially after work, if you have a job that leaves you hot and sweaty.
- Bathe or shower immediately after a workout.
- Apply talc or other powder to the groin area. This will help keep this area dry.
- Don't store damp clothing in a locker or gym bag.
- Wash workout clothes after each wearing.
- Sleep in the nude or in a nightshirt.
- Avoid antibacterial (deodorant) soaps.

An antifungal cream, powder or lotion like tolnaftate (brand name Tinactin) may also help relieve jock itch. It takes up to two weeks to work.

Testicular Cancer & Testicular Self-Exam

Cancer of the testicles, the primary make sex organs, accounts for only about 1 percent of all cancers in men. It is, though, the most common type of cancer in males aged 20 to 40, but can occur anytime after age 15. It strikes about 5,000 males a year. Often, only one testicle is affected. The cause of testicular cancer is not known. Risk factors, though, have been given. These are:

- Uncorrected undescended testicles in infants and young children. (Parents should see that their infant boys are checked at birth for the undescended testicles.)
- A family history of testicular cancer.
- Having an identical twin with testicular cancer.
- Viral infections.
- Injury to the scrotum.

Signs and Symptoms

In the early stages, testicular cancer may have no symptoms. When there are symptoms, they include:

- Small, painless lump in a testicle.
- Enlarged testicle.
- Feeling of heaviness in the testicle or groin.
- Pain in the testicle.
- A change in the way the testicle feels.
- Enlarged male breasts and nipples.
- Blood or fluid that accumulates suddenly in the scrotum.

Testicular cancer is curable 90 to 95 percent of the time if found and treated early. The testicle is surgically removed. Other things can further treat the disease:

- Chemotherapy.
- Radiation therapy.
- Surgically removing nearby lymph nodes if necessary.

The American Academy of Family Physicians Subcommittee for Male Patients recommends the teaching of testicular self-examination between the ages of 13 and 18. The testicles are located behind the penis and contained within the scrotum. They should be about the same size and feel smooth, rubbery and egg-shaped. The left one sometimes hangs lower than the right.

Testicular Cancer & Testicular self-Exam, continued

Questions to Ask

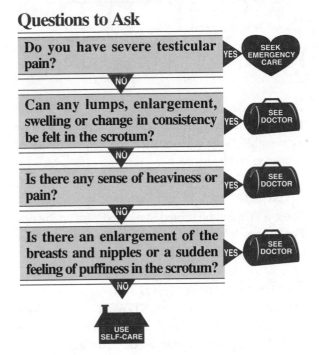

Perform Testicular Self-Exam (TSE) monthly or as recommended by your doctor.

Testicular Self-Exam (TSE)

Self-examination of the testicles is best performed when the scrotum is relaxed, after a warm bath or shower. This will also allow the testicles to drop down.

How to do TSE

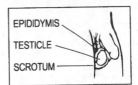
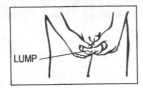

- Examine each testicle gently with both hands. The index and middle fingers should be placed underneath the testicle while the thumbs are placed on the top. Roll the testicle gently between the thumbs and fingers. One testicle may be larger than the other. This is normal.

- The epididymis is a cord-like structure on the top and back of the testicle that stores and transports the sperm. Do not confuse the epididymis with an abnormal lump.

- Feel for any abnormal lumps (about the size of a pea) on the front or the side of the testicle.

- These lumps are usually painless.

If you do find a lump, you should contact your doctor right away. The lump may be due to an infection and a doctor can decide the proper treatment. If the lump is not an infection, it is likely to be cancer. Remember that testicular cancer is highly curable, especially when detected and treated early. Testicular cancer almost always occurs in only one testicle and the other testicle is all that is needed for full sexual function.

Routine testicular self-exams are important, but they cannot substitute for a doctor's examination. Your doctor should examine your testicles when you have a physical exam. You can also ask your doctor to teach you the correct way to do a TSE.

chapter 20
SEXUALLY TRANSMITTED DISEASES (STDs)

Infections that pass from one person to another during sexual contact are known as sexually transmitted diseases (STDs). Sexual contact includes vaginal, anal and oral sex.

Sexually transmitted diseases include chlamydia, gonorrhea, syphilis and genital herpes. These are presented separately on pages 151 through 155. Acquired immune deficiency syndrome (AIDS) is often classified as a sexually transmitted disease, but can be passed through means other than sexual contact. So, though mentioned at times, it is not defined here. (See page 161 for information on "AIDS".) Note, though, that the self-care prevention tips on page 155 in this chapter can help prevent sexually acquired human immunodeficiency virus (HIV).

Basic Facts About STDs

Signs and Symptoms
Each STD has its own set of symptoms, but a discharge from the penis or vagina, pain when urinating (in males) and open sores or blisters in the genital area are typical of most STDs. Unfortunately, early stages of STDs often have no detectable symptoms. In addition, you can also have more than one STD at the same time. Gonorrhea and chlamydia, for example, are often picked up at the same time.

How STDs Spread
STDs are transmitted through intimate sexual contact.

Fast Response Counts
If you suspect you have an STD, see a doctor as soon as possible. Your sexual partner(s) should also be contacted and treated.

Treatment
Some STDs can be treated and cured with antibiotics. For others, such as herpes and acquired immune deficiency syndrome (AIDS), there is no cure.

Possible Complications
Depending on the infection, STDs can cause serious, long-term problems like birth defects, infertility, diseases of the brain, or, in the case of AIDS, death.

No "Shots" for Prevention
At present, no vaccines exist to prevent STDs.

Repeat Episodes
Once you've had an STD, you can get it again. You can't develop an immunity once you've been exposed.

Parents Don't Have to Know
A minor does not need parental consent to receive treatment for an STD.

[Note: Medical treatment, not self-care treatment, is necessary for sexually transmitted diseases. One exception is genital herpes for which many self-care remedies can help alleviate the discomfort that occurs with recurrent attacks. Self-Care Prevention Tips, however, should be followed to lower the risk for contracting STDs. (See page 155.)]

Chlamydia

Chlamydia is now the most common non-viral sexually transmitted disease in the United States. It affects more men and women than syphilis and gonorrhea combined. In fact, chances are that persons who have had these other sexually transmitted diseases (STDs) are playing host to chlamydia as well. Chlamydia can also accelerate the appearance of AIDS symptoms for persons infected with HIV (Human Immunodeficiency Virus).

Symptoms of chlamydia in men include burning or discomfort when urinating, a whitish discharge from the tip of penis and pain in the scrotum. In women, symptoms include slight yellowish-green vaginal discharge, vaginal irritation, a frequent need to urinate and pain when urinating. There can also be chronic abdominal pain and bleeding between menstrual periods.

These symptoms can, however, be so mild that they often go unnoticed. It is estimated that 75% of women and 25% of men who have chlamydia have no symptoms until complications set in. If they do appear, they usually do so two to four weeks after being infected. The only sure way to know whether or not you have chlamydia is to be tested. Doctors recommend that sexually active people who are not involved in a long-term, monogamous relationship be tested periodically. You should be aware, though, that the most reliable test for chlamydia is a tissue culture that is expensive and not widely available. For that reason, many doctors use a simpler slide test instead. A small amount of fluid is collected from the infected site with a cotton swab. Sometimes the results are available the same day of the test.

Anyone who has chlamydia should be treated with oral antibiotics such as tetracycline, erythromycin, or azithromycin. Doctors will treat the infected sexual partner even if he or she doesn't show any symptoms. Sex should be avoided until treatment is completed in both the person affected and in their sex partners. If left untreated, chlamydia can cause a variety of serious problems including infection and inflammation of the prostate and surrounding structures in men and pelvic inflammatory disease (PID) and infertility in women. Infants born to mothers who have chlamydia are likely to develop pneumonia or serious eye infections in the first several months of life as well as permanent lung damage later on.

Questions to Ask

For men: Do you have any of these problems:
- **A whitish discharge from the penis**
- **Burning or discomfort when urinating**
- **Pain and swelling in the scrotum?**

YES

NO

For women: Do you have these problems?
- **A yellowish-green vaginal discharge**
- **Frequent need to urinate**
- **Chronic abdominal pain**
- **Bleeding between menstrual periods**

YES

NO

Does your sexual partner have or do you suspect he or she might have a sexually transmitted disease? Does he or she have multiple sex partners?

YES

NO

Do you want to rule out the presence of chlamydia because you are considering a new sexual relationship, planning to get married or pregnant or for any other reason?

YES

NO

Use Self-care Prevention Tips on page 155.

Genital Herpes

Herpes simplex virus is spread by direct skin to skin contact from the site of infection to the contact site. Once you are infected, the virus remains with you forever. It causes symptoms, though, only during flare-ups. Symptoms include sores with blisters on the genital area and anus and sometimes on the thighs and buttocks. After a few days, the blisters break open and leave painful, shallow ulcers which can last from five days to three weeks. If infected for the first time, you may experience flu-like symptoms such as swollen glands, fever and body aches. Subsequent attacks are almost always much milder and much shorter in duration. These attacks may be triggered by emotional stress, fatigue, menstruation, other illnesses or even by vigorous sexual intercourse. Itching, irritation and tingling in the genital area may occur one to two days before the outbreak of the blisters or sores. (This period is called the prodrome.) Genital herpes is contagious during the prodrome when blisters are present and up to a week or two after they have disappeared. If a pregnant woman has an outbreak of genital herpes when her baby is due, a Caesarean section may need to be done so the baby does not get infected during delivery.

No cure exists for genital herpes. The prescription medication Zovirax, and self-help measures only treat herpes symptoms. (See "Self-Care Tips for Genital Herpes" in the next column.) Medication can be helpful during the first attack of genital herpes. Self-help remedies may be all that is necessary during recurrent episodes.

[Note: Herpes-like sores and blisters can be a side effect of taking certain prescription medicine in some people. One example is sulfa medications which are often used to treat urinary tract infections. Consult your doctor if you suspect this.]

Questions to Ask

Do you have sores and/or painful blisters on the genital area, anus or tongue and is this the first time you have had this? **YES**

NO

Did these sores appear only after taking a recently prescribed medicine? **YES**

NO

For persons who have already been diagnosed with genital herpes: Are you experiencing severe pain and blistering and/or are you having frequent attacks? **YES**

NO

For pregnant women only: Are these sores present and are you close to your delivery date? **YES**

NO

Have you had sexual relations with someone who had sores or blisters on their genital area, anus or tongue or had genital itching, irritation and tingling? **YES**

NO

Self-Care Tips for Genital Herpes

- Bathe the affected genital area twice a day with mild soap and water. Gently pat dry with a towel or use a hair dryer set on warm. Using Aveeno (colloidal oatmeal soap or bath treatments) may also be soothing.
- Take a hot bath if you can tolerate it. This may help to inactivate the virus and promote healing.
- Use sitz baths to soak the affected area. A sitz bath device fits over the toilet. You can get one at a medical supply store or at some pharmacies.

Genital Herpes, continued

- ☐ Apply ice packs on the genital area for 5-10 minutes. This may help relieve itching and inflammation.

- ☐ Wear loose fitting pants or skirts. Avoid wearing panty hose and tight fitting clothing. These could irritate the inflamed area. Wear cotton, not nylon, underwear.

- ☐ Squirt tepid water over the genital area while urinating. This may help decrease the pain.

- ☐ Take a mild pain reliever such as aspirin, acetaminophen, ibuprofen or naproxen sodium. *[Note: Do not give aspirin or any medication containing salicylates to anyone 19 years of age or younger unless directed by a physician due to its association with Reye's Syndrome, a potentially fatal condition.]*

- ☐ A local anesthetic ointment such as Lidocaine can help during the most painful part of an attack. (Check with your doctor before using.)

- ☐ Ask your doctor about using the oral anti-viral medicine acyclovir (brand name Zovirax).

- ☐ To avoid spreading the virus to your eyes, don't touch your eyes during an outbreak.

- ☐ Avoid sexual intercourse:
  - At the first sign of a herpes outbreak (this may be evident by the feeling of tingling and itching in the genital area which takes place before blisters are noticeable). Note, though, that herpes can be contracted without visible blisters because viral lesions may be present on the female's cervix or inside the male's urethra.
  - When active lesions are present
  - Two to three days after lesions have disappeared

Gonorrhea

Gonorrhea is one of the most common infectious diseases in the world. Often called "the clap", "dose", or "drip", it is caused by specific bacterium that is transmitted during vaginal, oral or anal sex. A newborn baby can also get gonorrhea during childbirth if its mother is infected. Gonorrhea can be symptom-free. In fact, about 60 to 80% of infected women have no symptoms.

The signs of gonorrhea can, however, show up within two to ten days after sexual contact with an infected person. In men, symptoms include pain at the tip of the penis, pain and burning during urination and a thick, yellow, cloudy penile discharge that gradually increases. In women, symptoms include mild itching and burning around the vagina, a thick, yellowish-green vaginal discharge, burning on urination and severe lower abdominal pain (usually within a week or so after their menstrual periods).

If ignored, gonorrhea can cause widespread infection and/or infertility. But, gonorrhea can be cured with specific antibiotics. Since many strains of gonorrhea are resistant to penicillin, your doctor will almost always use another medicine.

To treat gonorrhea successfully, you should heed the following:
- ☐ Take prescribed medications.
- ☐ To avoid re-infection, be sure that your sexual partner is also treated.
- ☐ Have follow-up cultures to determine if the treatment was effective.

Questions to Ask

For men only: Do you have any of these problems?
- **A discharge of pus from the penis**
- **Discomfort or pain when urinating**
- **Irritation and itching of the penis**
- **Pain during intercourse**

YES SEE DOCTOR

NO

flowchart continued in next column

Gonorrhea, continued

For women only: Do you have any of these problems?
- **Itching and burning around the vagina**
- **A vaginal discharge (this could be slight, cloudy or greenish-yellow in color)**
- **Burning or pain when urinating**
- **The need to urinate often**
- **Discomfort in the lower abdomen**
- **Abnormal bleeding from the vagina**

YES SEE DOCTOR

NO

Are you symptom-free, but suspicious of having contracted gonorrhea or another sexually transmitted disease from someone you suspect may be infected?

YES CALL DOCTOR

NO

Do you want to rule out the presence of a sexually transmitted disease because you have had multiple sex partners and you are considering a new sexual relationship, planning to get married or pregnant?

YES CALL DOCTOR

NO

Use Self-Care Prevention
Tips on page 155.

Syphilis

Syphilis is sometimes called "pox" or "bad blood". Left untreated, syphilis is one of the most serious sexually transmitted diseases, leading to heart failure, blindness, insanity or death. Syphilis can progress slowly through three stages over a period of many years. When detected early, however, syphilis can be cured. Be alert for the following symptoms:

Primary stage

A large, painless, ulcer-like sore known as a chancre occurs two to six weeks after infection and generally appears around the area of sexual contact. The chancre disappears within a few weeks.

Secondary stage

Within a month after the end of the primary stage, a widespread skin rash may appear cropping up on the palms of the hands, soles of the feet and sometimes around the mouth and nose. The rash commonly has small, red, scaling bumps that do not itch. Other types of rashes, swollen lymph nodes, fever and flu-like symptoms may also occur and small patches of hair may fall out of the scalp, beard, eyelashes and eyebrows.

Latent stage

Once syphilis reaches this stage, it may go unnoticed for years quietly damaging the heart, central nervous system, muscles and various other organs and tissues. The resulting effects are often fatal.

If you've been exposed to syphilis or have its symptoms, see a doctor or consult your county health department. For syphilis in its early stages, treatment consists of penicillin. If the disease has progressed further, you'll require three consecutive weekly injections. (If you're allergic to penicillin, you'll receive an alternative antibiotic taken orally for two to four weeks.) You should have a blood test 3,6 and 12 months after treatment to be sure the disease is completely cured.

Once treatment is complete, you're no longer contagious.

Syphilis, continued

Questions to Ask

Do you have a large, painless ulcer-like sore (chancre) in the genital area, anus or mouth? **YES**

NO ▼

Did you have such a sore several weeks to months ago that healed, but not experience flu-like symptoms (fever, headache, general ill-feeling) and/or a skin rash of small, red, scaling bumps that do not itch? **YES**

NO ▼

Are you suspicious of having contracted syphilis or another sexually transmitted disease from someone you suspect may be Infected? **YES**

NO ▼

Do you want to rule out the presence of syphilis or another sexually transmitted disease because you or your sex partner have had multiple sex partners and are considering a new sexual relationship, planning to get married or pregnant? **YES**

NO ▼

Use Self-Care Prevention Tips Listed Below.

Self-Care Prevention Tips

- There's only one way to guarantee you'll never get a sexually transmitted disease: Never have sex.
- Limiting your sexual activity to one person your entire life is a close second, provided your partner is also monogamous and does not have a sexually transmitted disease.
- Avoid sexual contact with persons whose health status and practices are not known.
- Don't have sex while under the influence of drugs or alcohol (except in a monogamous relationship in which neither partner is infected with an STD).
- Avoid sex if either partner has signs and symptoms of a genital tract infection.
- Discuss a new partner's sexual history with him or her before beginning a sexual relationship. (Be aware, though, that persons are not always honest about their sexual history.)
- **Latex condoms can reduce the spread of sexual diseases when used properly and carefully and for every sex act. They do not eliminate the risk entirely.**
- Both women and men should carry latex condoms and insist that they be used every time they have sexual relations.
- Using spermicidal foams, jellies, creams (especially those that contain Nonoxynol-9) and a diaphragm can offer additional protection when used with a condom. Use water-based lubricants such as K-Y Brand Jelly. Don't use oil-based or "petroleum" ones such as Vaseline. They can damage latex condoms.
- Wash the genitals with soap and water before and after sexual intercourse.
- Seek treatment for a sexually transmitted disease if you know your sex partner is infected.
- Ask your doctor to check for STDs every six months if you have multiple sex partners even if you don't have any symptoms.

chapter 21

DENTAL HEALTH

Abscess

A tooth abscess is formed when there is inflammation and/or infection in the bone and/or the tooth's canals. This generally occurs in a tooth that has a deep cavity, a very deep filling or one that has been injured. The pain caused by an abscessed tooth can be persistent, throbbing and severe. Other symptoms include fever, earache and swelling of the glands on one side of the face or neck. It can also cause a general ill feeling, bad breath and a foul taste in the mouth.

A tooth abscess is usually treated with either a root canal or by pulling the tooth. A root canal is done if the dentist thinks the tooth can be saved. The infection is first removed either through a hole drilled through the top of the tooth or through an incision made in the gums at the site of the infection. These measures relieve the pain and pressure caused by a tooth abscess. An antibiotic will also be prescribed.

Tooth abscesses, for the most part, can be prevented with regular dental care. This includes daily brushing (with a fluoride toothpaste) and flossing and regular dental check-ups and cleanings.

Questions to Ask

Do you have one or more of these problems with the toothache?
- **Continuous or throbbing pain**
- **Fever**
- **Earache**
- **Neck or jaw tenderness or swollen glands in the side where the tooth aches**
- **General ill feeling**
- **Bad breath and/or foul taste in the mouth**

YES SEE DOCTOR

NO

flowchart continued in next column

Does the pain come and go or only occur when you are eating or drinking? YES CALL DOCTOR

NO

 USE SELF-CARE

Self-Care Tips

☐ To reduce pain, take aspirin, acetaminophen, ibuprofen or naproxen sodium. *[Note: Do not give aspirin or any medication containing salicylates to anyone 19 years of age or younger unless directed by a physician, due to its association with Reye's Syndrome, a potentially fatal condition.]*

☐ Hold an ice pack on the jaw. This will relieve some of the pain.

☐ Never place a crushed aspirin on the tooth. Aspirin burns the gums and destroys tooth enamel. *[Note: Do not give aspirin or any medication containing salicylates to anyone 19 years of age or younger unless directed by a physician due to its association with Reye's Syndrome, a potentially fatal condition.]*

☐ Do not drink extremely hot or cold liquids.

☐ Do not chew gum.

☐ Avoid sweets and hot and spicy foods. A liquid diet may be necessary for a day or two until the pain subsides.

☐ Gargle with warm salt water every hour.

☐ See a dentist even if the pain subsides.

Broken Or Knocked Out Tooth

Your teeth are meant to last a lifetime. They can, however, be vulnerable to nicks, chips and strains. To protect your teeth from damage and injury, take these precautions:

- ☐ Don't chew ice, pens or pencils.
- ☐ Don't use your teeth to open paper clips or otherwise function as tools.
- ☐ If you smoke a pipe, don't bite down on the stem.
- ☐ If you grind your teeth at night, ask your dentist if you should be fitted for a bite plate to prevent tooth grinding.
- ☐ If you play contact sports like football or hockey, wear a protective mouth guard.
- ☐ Always wear a seat belt when riding in a car.
- ☐ Avoid sucking on lemons or chewing aspirin or vitamin C tablets. The acid wears away tooth enamel.

If a tooth does accidentally get knocked out, go to the dentist as soon as possible. Your dentist may be able to successfully put it back in. If this can be done within about a half an hour, there is a possibility that the interior pulp will survive. Even up to six hours, the outer tissue of the tooth may survive and allow successful re-attachment. There is little chance that the tooth can be put back in 24 hours after it has been knocked out. It is important to keep the tooth moist until you get to the dentist.

Questions to Ask

Has one or more teeth been broken or knocked out? YES SEEK EMERGENCY CARE

NO

USE SELF-CARE

[Note: See dentist as soon as possible. This is a dental emergency.]

Self-Care Tips

For a broken tooth:

- ☐ To reduce swelling, apply a cold compress to the area.
- ☐ Save any broken tooth fragments and take them to the dentist.

If your tooth has been knocked out:

- ☐ Rinse the tooth with clear water.
- ☐ If possible (and if you're alert), gently put it back in the socket or hold it under your tongue.
- ☐ Otherwise, put the tooth in a glass of milk or a wet cloth.
- ☐ If the gum is bleeding, hold a gauze pad, a clean handkerchief or tissue tightly in place over the wound.
- ☐ Try to get to a dentist within 30 minutes of the accident.

Periodontal Disease

Plaque build-up, crooked teeth, illness, poorly fitting dentures, trapped food particles and certain medications can irritate or destroy your gums. With good oral hygiene, however, you can prevent gum (periodontal) disease. If caught in the early stages, gum disease is easily treated. If ignored, the gums and supporting tissues wither and your teeth may loosen and fall out. Knowing the signs and symptoms of periodontal disease is important for early treatment. Pay attention to the following:

- ☐ Swollen red gums that bleed easily (a condition called gingivitis).
- ☐ Teeth that are exposed at the gum line (a sign that gums have pulled away from the teeth).
- ☐ Permanent teeth that are close or separating from each other.
- ☐ Bad breath and a foul taste in the mouth.
- ☐ Pus around the gums and teeth.

Periodontal disease should be treated by a periodontist, a dentist who specializes in this area of dentistry. Material called tartar or calculus (which is calcified plaque) can form even when normal brushing and flossing are done. The dentist or dental hygienist can remove tartar at regular intervals. When periodontitis (pockets of infection and areas of weakened bone) are established, the dentist can treat the problem with surgery or with a process known as "deep scaling".

Periodontal Disease, continued

Questions to Ask

Are one or more of the symptoms of gum disease present?
- **Swollen gums**
- **Gums that bleed easily**
- **Teeth exposed at the gum line**
- **Loose teeth**
- **Teeth separating from each other**
- **Pus around the gums and teeth**
- **Bad breath and/or a foul taste in the mouth**

YES

NO

Self-Care Tips

- Make sure to brush and floss your teeth regularly. Use a soft, rounded bristle toothbrush (unless your dentist has told you otherwise). Have your dentist or hygienist show you how to brush and floss your teeth correctly.
- Eat sugary foods infrequently. When you eat sweets, do so with meals, not in between meals.
- Finish a meal with cheese because this tends to neutralize acid formation.
- Include foods with good sources of vitamin A and vitamin C daily. (These two vitamins promote gum health.) You get vitamin A from cantaloupe, broccoli, spinach, winter squash, liver and dairy products fortified with vitamin A. Good vitamin C food sources include oranges, grapefruit, tomatoes, potatoes, green peppers and broccoli.

Temporomandibular Joint Syndrome (TMJ)

Temporomandibular joint (TMJ) syndrome occurs when the muscles, joints and ligaments of the jaw move out of alignment. Resulting symptoms include earaches, headaches, pain in the jaw area radiating to the face or the neck and shoulders, ringing in the ears or pain when opening and closing the mouth. These TMJ symptoms frequently mimic other conditions so the problem is often misdiagnosed. TMJ has a number of possible causes:

- Bruxism (grinding your teeth in your sleep).
- Sleeping in a way that mis-aligns the jaw or creates tension in the neck.
- Stress-induced muscle tension in the neck and shoulder.
- Incorrect or uneven bite.

TMJ may or may not require professional treatment. This should, however, be evaluated by a dentist. Many dentists specialize in the diagnosis and treatment of TMJ. They may prescribe anti-inflammatory medicine, tranquilizers or muscle relaxants for a short period of time, braces to correct the bite or a bite plate to wear when sleeping. Some doctors recommend surgery to correct TMJ, but you should get more than one opinion before consenting to a surgical remedy.

Questions to Ask

Are you unable to open or close your mouth because of severe pain?

YES

NO

Do you experience one or more of the following?
- **Inability to open the jaw completely**
- **Pain when you open your mouth widely**
- **Persistent symptoms of headache, earache or pain in the jaw area that is also felt in the face, neck or shoulders**
- **"Clicking" or "popping" sounds when you open your mouth and when you chew**

YES

NO

Temporomandibular Joint Syndrome (TMJ), continued

Self-Care Tips

If you have TMJ, you may be able to minimize symptoms in the following ways:

- ☐ Don't chew gum.
- ☐ Try not to open your jaw wide. This includes yawning, taking big bites out of triple-decker and submarine sandwiches or other difficult-to-eat foods).
- ☐ Massage the jaw area several times a day, first with your mouth open, then with your mouth closed.
- ☐ To help reduce muscle spasms that can cause pain, apply moist heat to the jaw area. (A washcloth soaked in warm water makes a convenient hot compress.)
- ☐ If stress is a factor, consider biofeedback and relaxation training.

Toothaches

The pain of a toothache can be felt in the tooth itself or in the region around the tooth. Most toothaches are usually the result of either a cavity or an infection beneath or around the gum of a tooth. Insufficient oxygen to the heart as experienced with angina or a heart attack can also cause a toothache. A toothache is common after having corrective dental work on a tooth, but this should not last longer than a week. (If it does, inform the dentist.)

Generally, toothaches can be prevented with regular visits to the dentist and daily self-care measures. Self-care includes proper daily brushing and flossing, good nutrition and using fluoridated water, toothpaste, rinse and supplement (if prescribed).

Tell your dentist if you notice any of the following. (They may lead to a toothache if left unchecked.)

- ☐ Sensitivity to hot, cold or sweet foods
- ☐ Brown spots or little holes on a tooth
- ☐ A change in your bite - the way your teeth fit together
- ☐ Loose teeth in an adult

Questions to Ask

Do you have any of these problems with the tooth pain?
- **Gnawing pain in the lower teeth or neck**
- **Chest discomfort beneath the breast bone**
- **Pain that travels to or is felt in the arm**
- **Sweating**

NO

Are any of the following symptoms present?
- **Fever**
- **Red, swollen or bleeding gums**
- **Swollen face**
- **Foul breath even after thorough brushing and flossing**
- **Constant toothache even when sleeping at night**
- **Toothache only when eating or just after eating**

NO

Self-Care Tips

- ☐ To reduce discomfort, take aspirin or other mild pain reliever.
- ☐ Hold an ice pack on the jaw. This will relieve some of the pain.
- ☐ Never place a crushed aspirin on the tooth. Aspirin burns the gums and destroys tooth enamel.
- ☐ Do not drink extremely hot or cold liquids.
- ☐ Do not chew gum.
- ☐ Avoid sweets, soft drinks and hot and spicy foods. (These can irritate cavities and increase pain.) It may be best not to eat at all until you see your doctor.
- ☐ Gargle with warm salt water every hour.
- ☐ For a cavity, pack it with a piece of sterile cotton soaked in oil of cloves (available at pharmacies.)
- ☐ See a dentist even if the pain subsides.

SECTION III
Major Medical Conditions

Introduction

Section III presents 15 chronic illnesses. Each of the conditions is divided into 3 parts.

- Information about the condition.
- Signs and symptoms of the condition.
- Care and treatment for the condition.

Unlike the 75 common health problems in Section II, which you may be able to treat with Self-Care Tips alone, these 15 chronic medical conditions need a doctor's diagnosis and medical treatment from health care professionals. Still, there will be things you will need to do to take care of yourself, if you have one or more of these conditions.

chapter 22
CHRONIC ILLNESSES

AIDS

AIDS stands for Acquired Immune Deficiency Syndrome. It is thought to be caused by the human immunodeficiency virus (HIV). This virus destroys the body's immune system, leaving the person unable to fight certain types of infection or cancer. The virus also attacks the central nervous system, causing mental and neurological problems.

The virus is carried in body fluids such as semen, vaginal secretions, breast milk and blood (including menstrual blood).

Certain activities are likely to promote contracting HIV. High-risk activities include:

▭ Unprotected* anal, oral and/or vaginal sex except in a monogamous relationship in which neither partner is infected with HIV. Particularly high risk situations are having sex:
  • When drunk or high.
  • With multiple or casual sex partners.
  • With a partner who has had multiple or casual sex partners.
  • With a partner who has used drugs by injection or is bisexual.
  • When you or your partner has signs and symptoms of a genital tract infection.

* Unprotected means without using condoms alone or with other latex or polyurethane barriers. When used correctly every time and for every sex act, these provide protection from HIV. Though not 100% effective, they will reduce the risk. Male latex condoms are preferred. The Reality female condom also offers protection, especially when used with a male condom.

▭ Sharing needles and/or "the works" when injecting any kind of drugs.
▭ Pregnancy and delivery if the mother is infected with HIV. This can put the child at risk.
▭ Having had blood transfusions, especially before 1985, unless tested negative for HIV.

There is some concern about the risk of getting HIV from an infected doctor, dentist or patient. There are almost no cases of health professionals passing HIV to a patient. Patient to health professional transmission has been more noted. Measures are being proposed and required by medical and dental associations to decrease these possible risks, even though they are extremely low.

Blood screening tests are also done on donated blood which makes it highly unlikely that you'd get HIV from current blood transfusions. You cannot get HIV from donating blood or from casual contact such as:

▭ Touching, holding hands or hugging.
▭ A cough, sneeze, tears or sweat.
▭ An animal or insect bite.
▭ A toilet seat.
▭ Using a hot tub or swimming.

Screening tests for HIV are available through doctors' offices, clinics and health departments. A small sample of your blood is tested for antibodies to the HIV virus. If these antibodies are present, you test positive for and are considered infected with HIV. It could take as long as six months from exposure to the virus for these antibodies to show up. The most common reason for a false negative test is when a person gets tested before HIV antibodies have formed. If you test positive for HIV, a second type of blood test is done to confirm it. HIV/AIDS symptoms may not show up for as long as eight to eleven years after a person is infected with the virus.

Home collection testing kits, such as CONFIDE and *Home Access* are available over-the-counter. Follow package directions. The results are kept anonymous and confidential.

AIDS, continued

Signs and Symptoms

Early symptoms of HIV/AIDS:

- Fatigue.
- Loss of appetite.
- Chronic diarrhea.
- Weight loss.
- Persistent dry cough.
- Fever.
- Night sweats.
- Swollen lymph nodes.

Persons with AIDS fall prey to many diseases such as skin infections, fungal infections, tuberculosis, pneumonia and cancer. These "opportunistic" infections are what lead to death in an AIDS victim. When HIV invades the brain cells, it leads to forgetfulness, impaired speech, trembling and seizures.

Prevention

Some day, a cure for AIDS may exist. For now, prevention is the only protection. Take these steps to avoid contracting HIV:

- Unless you are in a long-term, monogamous relationship, use male latex condoms every time you have sex. The spermicide, Nonoxynol-9, may inactivate the virus. Use the spermicide with a male latex condom, not alone.
- Don't have sex with people who are at high risk for contracting HIV. These have been noted to be:
  - Homosexual or bisexual men especially with multiple sex partners or who use illegal intravenous drugs.
  - Heterosexual partners of persons infected or exposed to HIV.
  - Persons who have had multiple blood transfusions, especially before 1985, unless tested negative.
- Don't have sex with more than one person.

- Ask specific questions about your partner's sexual past, i.e., have they had many partners or unprotected (no condom) sex? Do not be afraid to ask if they have been tested for HIV and if the results were positive or negative.
- Don't have sex with anyone who you know or suspect has had multiple partners. (If you've had sex with someone you suspect is HIV positive, see your doctor).
- Don't share needles and/or "the works" with anyone. This includes not only illegal drugs such as heroin but steroids, insulin, etc. Don't have sex with people who use or have used intravenous drugs.
- Don't share personal items that have blood on them, such as razors.

Treatment and Care

Current treatments for AIDS include:

- Medications: AZT, DDI, DDC, D4T, 3TC with AZT. These slow the virus but do not destroy it. A newer class of medicines called protease inhibitors may help keep HIV from growing. Combinations of medicines are often used.
- Taking measures to reduce the risk of getting infections and diseases. Get adequate rest, proper nutrition and take vitamin supplements as suggested by your doctor.
- Emotional support.
- Treating the "opportunistic" infections that occur, for example:
  - Antibiotics such as Bactrim or Septra for pneumonia.
- Radiation therapy and surgery have been used in the treatment of some patients.

AIDS is under intensive study and research. Better forms of treatment and a vaccine are being researched world wide. A single vaccine to protect against AIDS is not very likely, though, because HIV quickly creates new strains of the virus.

Alzheimer's Disease

Mysterious and frustrating, Alzheimer's afflicts nearly four million Americans, about 10 percent of the population over age 65, and over 45 percent of those over age of 85. (In rare instances, Alzheimer's strikes earlier than 65).

No one knows what causes Alzheimer's disease. Some research hints that a virus or infectious agent is the culprit. Others point to brain chemical deficits, a genetic predisposition and/or environmental toxins. Nevertheless, the end result is the death of brain cells that control intellect (the way your brain receives and processes information).

Signs and Symptoms

Alzheimer's Disease has a gradual onset. The signs and symptoms may progress in stages. How quickly they occur varies from person to person. The disease may, however, eventually leave its victims totally unable to care for themselves.

Stage One

- Forgetfulness.
- Disorientation of time and place.
- Increasing inability to do routine tasks.
- Impairment in judgement.
- Lessening of initiative.
- Lack of spontaneity.
- Depression and fear.

Stage Two

- Increasing forgetfulness.
- Increasing disorientation.
- Wandering.
- Restlessness and agitation, especially at night.
- Repetitive actions.
- Muscle twitching and/or convulsions may develop.

Stage Three

- Disorientation.
- Inability to recognize either themselves or other people.
- Speech impairment (may not be able to speak at all).
- Develop need to put everything into their mouths.
- Develop need to touch everything in sight.
- Become emaciated.
- Complete loss of control of all body functions.

[Note: The stages very often overlap.]

Treatment and Care

If someone you care about shows signs of Alzheimer's disease, see that they get medical attention to confirm (or rule out) the diagnosis. Not everything that looks like Alzheimer's is Alzheimer's. There are many diseases or other problems that can cause dementia (severe problems with memory and thinking). These include:

- Brain tumors.
- Blood clots in the brain.
- Severe vitamin B12 deficiency.
- Hypothyroidism.
- Depression.
- Some medicine side effects.

(Unlike Alzheimer's, these problems can be treated).

There is no known cure for Alzheimer's Disease. Because no specific treatment or medicine exists to slow the steady deterioration that typifies Alzheimer's, good planning or medical and social management are necessary to help both the victim and care-givers cope with the symptoms and maintain the quality of life for as long as possible. It's especially helpful to put structure in the life of someone who's in the early stages of Alzheimer's. Some suggestions include:

- Maintain daily routines.
- Post reminders on an oversized and prominently displayed calendar.

Alzheimer's Disease, continued

- Make "to do" lists of daily tasks for the person with Alzheimer's to complete, and ask him or her to check them off as they're completed.
- Put things in their proper places after use, to help the person with Alzheimer's find things when he or she needs them.
- Post safety reminders (like "turn off the stove") at appropriate places throughout the house.
- Also, see that the person with Alzheimer's eats well-balanced meals, goes for walks with family members, and otherwise continues to be as active as possible.

Most medication therapies currently being used are experimental. Two prescription medications, Cognex, and Aricept, may help with memory in some persons with the early stage of Alzheimer's Disease. Sometimes medications to treat depression, paranoia and agitation, etc. can minimize symptoms, but they will not necessarily improve memory.

At late stages, providing a safe environment is of utmost importance. Alzheimer's victims should wear identification bracelets or necklaces so they can be identified should they be separated from their home environment. Seeking adult foster care or nursing home care for those who require supervision or medical management may be necessary.

Care-givers of Alzheimer's victims should also be given "care." They must deal with a number of financial, social, physical and emotional issues. Care for care-givers can be provided by professionals of home care, day care, respite care, service programs and self-help groups.

Angina

Angina is a common term shortened for the medical term "angina pectoris". The word angina itself means pain; pectoris means chest. Angina is the chest pain or discomfort brought on by decreased circulation in the heart and heart muscle itself. It results from a shortage of oxygen and other nutrients to any part of the heart muscle.

Signs and Symptoms

- Squeezing pressure, heaviness, or mild ache in the chest (usually behind the breastbone).
- Aching in a tooth accompanied by this squeezing pressure or heaviness in the chest.
- Aching into the neck muscles or jaw.
- Aching into one or both arms in whole or in part.
- Aching into the back.
- A feeling of gas in the upper abdomen and lower chest.
- A feeling that you're choking.
- Paleness and sweating.

These symptoms may not be extreme so are often neglected. It is better for you to report an episode of angina to your doctor than not to, even if you might feel foolish later if something minor is the cause. Episodes of angina are usually associated with:

- Anger or excitement.
- Emotional shock.
- Physical work in which the discomfort goes away when the work is stopped.
- Waking up at night with discomfort.
- Arm use.

In all of these situations, there is relief from the distress when the activity is stopped.

Many people who experience angina for the first time fear they're having a heart attack. Here's why angina and heart attack are mistaken for each other:

- Both can be caused by a buildup of fatty plaque (atherosclerosis) in the heart arteries (coronary arteries). These plaques cause a decrease in flow to the heart muscle beyond the partial obstruction. In both, the pain is felt in the chest and may spread to both arms, shoulders, or neck.
- Both may be brought on by physical exertion
- Both are most prevalent in men who are 50 and older and women who are past menopause

Angina, continued

But there are key differences, too:

- A heart attack results in a damaged or injured heart muscle, angina does not. Rather, anginal pain is a warning sign of a potential heart attack.
- The pain indicates that the heart muscle isn't getting enough blood.
- Rest or nitroglycerin relieves angina, but not a heart attack.

A doctor can generally diagnose angina as stable or unstable, based on your description of the painful episode, but he or she many need to confirm it with a stress test (a measurement of heart function taken while you exercise on a treadmill). Unstable angina, a symptom of coronary artery disease, requires immediate attention. This serious medical condition affects many Americans, some of whom may not know they have heart disease. Although unstable angina can be a precursor to heart attack, prompt treatment can lower the risk of death or serious cardiac events.

Factors like high blood pressure, obesity, diabetes, high cholesterol, smoking, or a family history of atherosclerotic heart disease increase the odds of angina.

Treatment and Care

Seek emergency care for any chest pain which is suspicious for angina. Contact your physician or a cardiologist who should insist on close follow-up, appropriate studies to diagnose your condition, and therapy to treat it. The keystones to treatment are:

- Appropriate medicine such as one to control high blood pressure; nitroglycerin or other medication to temporarily dilate or widen the coronary arteries which ease blood flow to the heart. Nitroglycerin takes effect within a minute or two.
- Daily physical exercise for endurance, preferably prescribed just for you by an exercise physiologist to whom a cardiologist has referred you. Exercise must be maintained below the onset of any discomfort. It may not be applicable at all for some individuals.

- Don't smoke. Nicotine in cigarettes constricts the arteries and prevents proper blood flow.
- Avoid large, heavy meals. Instead, eat lighter meals throughout the day.
- Rest after eating, or engage in some quiet activity.
- Minimize exposure to cold, windy weather.
- Lower your cholesterol level, if high, by eating a low saturated fat diet and/or taking lipid (fat) lowering medication, if necessary and prescribed.
- Avoid sudden engagement in rather severe exercise or other physical stress.
- Avoid anger and frustration whenever possible.

Arthritis

Arthritis robs some 40 million Americans of their freedom of movement by breaking down the protective cartilage in the joints. By destroying cartilage, arthritis results in pain and decreased movement.

Many forms of arthritis exist. Three of the most common are osteoarthritis, rheumatoid arthritis, and ankylosing spondylitis.

Osteoarthritis is a painful degeneration of the cartilage in the weight-bearing and frequently used joints. As far as researchers can tell, this kind of arthritis is typically brought on by genetics, activity, and wear and tear on the joints. It can also follow an injury to the joint. Osteoarthritis usually affects older people and is the most common type of arthritis.

Rheumatoid arthritis (RA) is caused by a chronic inflammation of the fingers, wrists, ankles, elbows, and/ or knees, causing pain, swelling, and tenderness. Morning stiffness lasting longer than an hour is very common. RA affects women more often than men, striking in their thirties and forties.

Ankylosing spondylitis generally affects young men between the ages of 15 and 45 and is characterized by a stiff backbone, accompanied by low back pain.

Signs and Symptoms

Symptoms of arthritis, therefore, depend upon the type of arthritis that is present. Symptoms generally include:

- Stiffness.
- Swelling in one or more joints.
- Deep, aching pain in a joint.
- Any pain associated with movement of a joint.
- Tenderness, warmth, or redness in afflicted joints.
- Fever, weight loss, or fatigue that accompanies joint pain.

Treatment and Care

If your doctor does diagnose arthritis, he or she may prescribe medication (usually aspirin or a non-steroidal anti-inflammatory medicine), rest, heat or cold treatment, and some physical therapy or exercise, depending on what kind of arthritis you have. The goal is to reduce pain and improve joint mobility.

Among those treatments, exercise is perhaps the most important, whether it be some form of stretching, isometrics, or simple endurance exercise. Low-impact exercise seems to provide both physical relief and psychological benefits. For example, it prevents the muscles from shrinking, while inactivity encourages both loss of muscle tone and bone deterioration. Too much exercise, however, will cause more pain in those with rheumatoid arthritis or osteoarthritis. So if you have arthritis, consult your physician, a physical therapist, or a physiatrist (a doctor who specializes in rehabilitative treatment) to assist you in developing an exercise program.

One form of exercise that's effective and soothing is hydrotherapy, or movement done in water. It allows freedom of movement and puts less stress on the joints because nearly all of the body weight is supported by the water. Doctors highly recommend swimming, too. But remember, hydrotherapy, or any form of exercise, should never produce pain. One message that can't be emphasized enough is "Go easy". If you begin to hurt, stop and rest or apply ice packs.

The following exercise suggestions may provide relief:

- Choose exercise routines that use all affected joints.
- Keep movements gradual, slow, and gentle.
- If a joint is inflamed, don't exercise it.
- Don't overdo it. Allow yourself sufficient rest.
- Concentrate on freedom of movement, especially in the water, and be patient.

Cancer

Cancer refers to a broad group of diseases in which body cells grow out of control and are or become malignant (harmful).

Cancer is the second leading cause of death in the United States (heart disease is first). Current estimates say that 30 percent of all Americans will develop some kind of cancer in their lifetimes. The most common forms are cancer of the skin, lungs, colon and rectum, breast, prostate, urinary tract, and uterus.

Exactly what causes all cancers has not yet been found. Evidence suggests, however, that cancer could result from complex interactions of viruses, a person's genetic make-up, their immune status and their exposure to other risk factors that may promote cancer.

These risk factors include:

- Exposure to the sun's ultraviolet rays, nuclear radiation, X-rays, and radon.
- Use of tobacco and/or alcohol (for some cancers).
- Use of certain medicines such as DES (a synthetic estrogen).
- Polluted air and water.
- Dietary factors such as a high fat diet, specific food preservatives, namely nitrates and nitrites; char-broiling and char-grilling meats.
- Exposure to a variety of chemicals such as asbestos, benzenes, VC (vinyl chloride), wood dust, some ingredients of cigarette smoke, etc.).

Cancer, continued

Signs and Symptoms

Symptoms of cancer depend on the type of cancer, the stage that it is in, and whether or not it has spread to other parts of the body (metastasis). The following signs and symptoms should always be brought to your doctor's attention because they could be warning signals of cancer:

- Any change in bladder or bowel habits.
- A lump or thickening in the breast, testicles or anywhere else.
- Unusual vaginal bleeding or rectal discharge or any unusual bleeding.
- Persistent hoarseness or nagging cough.
- A sore that doesn't heal.
- Noticeable change in a wart or mole.
- Indigestion or difficulty swallowing.

Treatment and Care

Cancer is not necessarily fatal and is, in many cases, curable. Early detection and proper treatment increase your chances for surviving cancer. Early detection is more likely if you:

- Know the above warning signs for cancer and report any of these warning signs to your doctor if they occur
- Do regular self-examination such as monthly breast self-examination if you are a woman, (see page 138) and a monthly testicular self-exam monthly or as directed by your doctor if you are a man (see page 149). *[Note: Men can also get breast cancer and should check with their doctor for signs to look for.]*
- Look at yourself in the mirror for any noticeable changes in warts or moles or for any wounds that have not healed
- Ask your doctor to perform routine tests that can help detect early signs of cancer. See "Tests and What They are For" on page 16 and "Common Health Tests" on page 17.

If and when cancer is diagnosed, treatment will depend on the type of cancer present, the stage it is in, and your body's response to treatment.

Cancer treatment generally includes one or more of the following:

- Surgery to remove the cancerous tumor(s) and
- clear any obstruction to vital passageways caused by the cancer.
- Radiation therapy.
- Chemotherapy.
- Possibly immunotherapy, hormonal therapy, or bone-marrow transplant.

Prevention

Moreover, measures can be taken to lower the risk for certain forms of cancer:

Dietary:

- Reduce the intake of total dietary fat to no more than 30% of total calories and reduce the intake of saturated fat to less than 10% of total calories
- Eat more fruits, vegetables, and whole grains, especially:
  - Broccoli and other cabbage family vegetables including cabbage and brussel sprouts. These contain cancer-fighting chemical, such as sulforaphane antioxidants.
  - Deep yellow-orange fruits and vegetables such as canteloupe, peaches, tomatoes, carrots, sweet potatoes, squash and very dark green vegetables like spinach, greens and broccoli for their beta-carotene content.
  - Strawberries, citrus fruits, broccoli and green peppers for vitamin C.
  - Whole grain breads, cereals, fresh fruits and vegetables and legumes for their dietary fiber content.
- Consume salt-cured, salt-pickled, and smoked foods only in moderation.
- Drink alcoholic beverages only in moderation, if at all.

Cancer, continued

Lifestyle:

- Do not smoke, use tobacco products or inhale second hand smoke.
- Limit your exposure to known carcinogens such as asbestos, radon, and other workplace chemicals as well as pesticides and herbicides.
- Have X-rays only when necessary.
- Limit your exposure to the sun's ultraviolet (UV) rays, sun lamps and tanning booths. Protect your skin from the sun's UV rays with sunscreen (applied frequently and containing a sun protection factor (SPF) of 15 or higher) and protective clothing (sun hats, long sleeves, etc.).
- Reduce stress. Emotional stress may weaken the immune system that is relied on to fight off stray cancer cells.

Chronic Fatigue Syndrome

Chronic fatigue syndrome has sometimes been called "yuppie flu" because its victims are often well-educated professionals in their twenties, thirties, and forties. Many are women. Until about 1983, doctors knew next to nothing about this malady and its exact cause is still unknown. Some researchers believed it was caused by the Epstein-Barr virus, whereas others suggest its cause could be a virus that has not yet been identified. Most experts now lean toward a theory of multiple causes.

Signs and Symptoms

Symptoms of chronic fatigue syndrome are:

- Fatigue for at least six months.
- Sore throat.
- Swollen glands.
- Low-grade fever.
- Headaches.
- Depression.
- Muscle aches.
- Mild weight loss.
- Short-term memory problems.
- Sleep disturbances (insomnia or hypersomnia).
- Confusion, difficulty thinking, inability to concentrate.

Unfortunately, these symptoms could signal any one of many diseases, and chronic fatigue syndrome can be diagnosed, therefore, only after other illnesses, such as AIDS, tuberculosis, chronic inflammatory diseases, auto-immune diseases, such as lupus, or psychiatric illnesses have been ruled out. There are no specific laboratory tests as yet, that can diagnose the syndrome.

For some, the symptoms are so debilitating that a normal working life is impossible. Yet others experience only a vague sense of feeling ill. In some cases, symptoms never let up, while in others they come and go.

Treatment/Care

Until more is known, people with chronic fatigue syndrome are encouraged to do the following:

- Get plenty of rest.
- Learn to manage stress.
- Take good care of their general health.
- Try to lead as normal a life as possible.
- Join a support group of others who have this problem.

Medicines may be prescribed to relieve pain and muscle aches and control fever such as acetaminophen, aspirin, ibuprofen, naproxen sodium or prescription, non-steroidal, anti-inflammatory medicine. Anti-depressant medicine may also be prescribed. A gradual exercise program, if tolerated, may also be beneficial.

Coronary Heart Disease

The coronary arteries supply blood to the heart muscle. When they became narrowed or blocked (usually by fatty deposits and or blood clots), the heart muscle can be damaged. This is coronary heart disease. Two conditions of coronary heart disease are "angina pectoris" (See angina on page 164), and acute myocardial infarction (heart attacks). Every day, about 4,000 Americans have heart attacks, one every 20 seconds. And each year, nearly 600,000 people die of coronary artery disease, making it the nation's number one killer. Fortunately, heart disease claims fewer and fewer lives each year, thanks to advances in medical treatment of heart disease and growing public awareness of the benefits of exercise and good nutrition. Prevention is of utmost importance.

Prevention

To avoid coronary heart disease, the American Heart Association suggests the following steps:

- ☐ Have your blood pressure checked regularly. High blood pressure can increase the risk of atherosclerosis. To control high blood pressure, follow your doctor's advice.
- ☐ If you smoke, quit. Nicotine constricts blood flow to the heart, decreases oxygen supply to the heart, and seems to play a significant role in the development of coronary artery disease.
- ☐ Be aware of the signs and symptoms for diabetes, which is associated with atherosclerosis. Follow his or her advice if you have diabetes. (See Diabetes on page 170).
- ☐ Maintain a normal body weight. (People who are obese are more prone to atherosclerosis, high blood pressure, and diabetes, and therefore coronary heart disease).
- ☐ Eat a diet low in saturated fats and cholesterol. (Saturated fats are found in meats, dairy products with fat, hydrogenated vegetable oils and some tropical oils, like coconut and palm kernel oils). High-saturated fat, high-cholesterol diets contribute to the fatty sludge that accumulates inside artery walls.
- ☐ Reduce your intake of salt if you are "salt-sensitive." Salt sensitive persons' blood pressure goes up if they eat too much salt.
- ☐ Get some form of aerobic exercise at least three times a week for 20 minutes at a time. Sitting around hour after hour, day after day, week in and week out with no regular physical activity may cause circulation problems later in life and contributes to atherosclerosis. Start new exercise programs gradually. Report symptoms of chest pain and/or shortness of breath to your doctor.
- ☐ Reduce the harmful effects of stress by practicing relaxation techniques and improving your outlook on daily events. Stress has been linked to elevated blood pressure, among other health problems.
- ☐ Get regular medical checkups.

- ☐ Know the signs of a heart attack so you can get immediate medical attention if necessary, before it's too late. The signs of a heart attack are:
  - Chest discomfort or pressure lasting several minutes or longer.
  - Discomfort or pressure that spreads to the shoulder, neck, arm, and jaw.
  - Nausea or vomiting associated with chest pain.
  - A cold sweat.
  - Difficulty breathing.
  - Faintness or dizziness.
  - Stomach upset.
  - A sense of impending disaster.

Treatment and Care

If you think you're having a heart attack, get to a hospital as quickly as possible. A clot dissolving injection can be given to reduce the risk of mortality and severity of damage to the heart muscle if given within four hours. Other emergency procedures can also prevent damage to the heart muscle.

The type of care following a heart attack will depend on the amount of damage done to the heart muscle which can be assessed by specific medical tests and procedures. Your doctor will determine the course of treatment. This could include any or many of the following:

- ☐ Medication (cardiac, blood pressure, cholesterol lowering medicines, etc.).
- ☐ Hospitalization for treatment and recovery from the heart attack.
- ☐ Cardiac rehabilitation for lifestyle changes including: Smoking cessation, weight loss, low-fat, cholesterol-controlling diet, behavior modification and stress management relaxation techniques.
- ☐ Surgery if indicated: Angioplasty, coronary artery bypass grafts, etc.
- ☐ Long-term maintenance and medical follow-up.

Diabetes

Diabetes is a condition which results when a person's body doesn't make any insulin, or enough insulin, or doesn't use insulin the right way. Insulin is a hormone made in the pancreas gland that helps your cells use blood sugar for energy. When insulin is in short supply, the glucose (sugar) in the blood can become dangerously high. That's why someone who is diabetic may have to take insulin by injection, or pills by mouth to help the body secrete more of its own insulin or make better use of the insulin it does secrete. Some diabetics, however, require no medication. All persons with diabetes must follow a controlled diet and exercise regularly to prevent their blood sugar from getting too high.

There are two (2) forms of diabetes:

Type 1 - (sometimes called insulin-dependent diabetes mellitus (IDDM) or juvenile diabetes) is more severe and usually shows up before the age of 30 (but may occur at any age). Insulin injections are essential as well as dietary control and exercise.

Type 2 - (sometimes called non-insulin dependent diabetes mellitus (NIDDM) or adult-onset diabetes) is less severe, usually affecting persons who are forty (40) years of age or older and overweight. This type is most often treated with diet and exercise and sometimes oral medicine. Occasional insulin injections may be required as well.

Diabetes can contribute to hardening of the arteries, strokes, kidney failure, blindness, and gangrene.

Signs and Symptoms

The American Diabetes Association uses the acronyms DIABETES and CAUTION to help identify the warning signs of diabetes.
- Drowsiness.
- Itching.
- A family history of diabetes.
- Blurred vision.
- Excessive weight.
- Tingling, numbness, or pain in extremities.
- Easy fatigue.
- Skin infection, slow healing of cuts and scratches, especially on the feet.

Other signs are:
- Constant urination.
- Abnormal thirst.
- Unusual hunger.
- The rapid loss of weight.
- Irritability.
- Obvious weakness and fatigue.
- Nausea and vomiting.

You don't necessarily have to experience all of these warning signs to be diabetic; only one or two may be present. Some people show no warning signs whatsoever and find out they're diabetic after a routine blood test. If you have a family history of diabetes, you should be especially watchful of the signs and symptoms above. If you notice any of these signs, report them to your doctor. Being overweight increases your risk significantly. A diet high in sugar and low in fiber may increase your risk if you are prone to developing diabetes. Pregnancy can trigger diabetes in some women.

Treatment and Care

Treatment for diabetes will depend on the type and severity of the disorder. Both forms, however, require a treatment plan that maintains normal, steady blood sugar levels. This can be accomplished by:
- Proper dietary measures that give prescribed amounts of protein, fat, and carbohydrates, are set up in regular meals adequate in intake of dietary fiber, and promote weight reduction, if necessary.
- Exercise.
- Medicine: Oral hypoglycemic agents, pills, or insulin injections, if necessary.

With either type of diabetes, routine care and follow up treatment is important. Careful control of blood sugar levels can allow a person with diabetes to lead a normal, productive life. Persons who are genetically predisposed to diabetes should watch their weight, control their eating habits, and exercise regularly to reduce their risk of getting the disease.

Diverticulosis

No one is sure why, but sometimes small sac-like pockets protrude from the wall of the colon. This is called diverticulosis. Increased pressure within the intestines seems to be responsible. The pockets (called diverticuli) can fill with intestinal waste.

Sometimes, though, the intestinal pouches become inflamed, in which case the condition is called diverticulitis.

Many older persons have diverticulosis. The digestive system becomes sluggish as a person ages. Things that increase the risk for diverticulosis include:

- Not eating enough dietary fiber. Diverticulosis is common in nations where fiber intake is low.
- Continual use of medicines that slow bowel action. (Examples: Painkillers and anti-depressants).
- Overuse of laxatives.
- Having family members who have diverticulosis.
- Having gallbladder disease.
- Being obese.

Signs and Symptoms

In most cases, diverticulosis causes no discomfort. When there are symptoms they are usually:

- Tenderness, mild cramping or a bloated feeling usually on the lower left side of the abdomen.
- Sometimes constipation or diarrhea.
- Occasionally, bright red blood in the stools.

With diverticulitis, you can experience severe abdominal pain, feel nauseous, and have a fever. The pain is made worse with a bowel movement. If these things occur, you should see your doctor.

Treatment and Care

Diverticular disease can't be cured, but you can reduce the discomfort, and prevent complications. Eat a diet high in fiber throughout life. You can add more fiber to your diet with fresh fruits and vegetables, and whole-grain foods. Check with your doctor about adding wheat bran to your diet. These pass through the system quickly, decreasing pressure in the intestines. Do, however, avoid corn, seeds, and foods with seeds like figs. These are easily trapped in the troublesome pouches.

You should also drink 1-1/2 to 2 quarts of water every day. Avoid the regular use of laxatives that make your bowel muscles contract such as Ex-Lax. In fact, you should consult your doctor before taking any laxatives. If you are not able to eat a high-fiber diet, ask your doctor about taking bulk-producing laxatives like Metamucil. These are not habit-forming. Try, too, not to strain when you have bowel movements. Finally, get regular exercise.

High Blood Pressure

High blood pressure isn't like a toothache, a bruise, or constipation. Nothing hurts, looks discolored, or fails to work. Usually, people with high blood pressure experience no discomfort or outward signs of trouble. Yet high blood pressure (hypertension) is a killer, a silent killer. Directly or indirectly, high blood pressure accounts for nearly a million deaths a year. Uncontrolled, high blood pressure increases the odds that you'll have a heart attack, a stroke, or kidney failure or loss of vision.

High blood pressure happens when your blood moves through your arteries at a higher pressure than normal. The heart is actually straining to pump blood through the arteries. This isn't healthy because:

- It promotes hardening of the arteries (atherosclerosis). Hardened, narrowed arteries may not be able to carry the amount of blood the body's organs need.
- Blood clots can form or lodge in a narrowed artery. (This could cause a stroke or heart attack).
- The heart can become enlarged. (This could result in congestive heart failure).

High Blood Pressure, continued

More than half of all older adults have high blood pressure. About fifty percent of all people who have it don't know it. Worse yet, many people who know their blood pressure is dangerously high are doing nothing to try to control it. And for 90 percent of those affected, there is no known cause. When this is the case, it is called primary or essential hypertension. When high blood pressure results from another medical disorder or a medicine it is referred to as secondary hypertension. In these cases (about 10% of total), when the root cause is corrected, blood pressure usually goes back to normal.

Detection

How's your blood pressure? Blood pressure is normally measured with a blood pressure cuff placed on the arm. The numbers on the gauge measure your blood pressure in millimeters of mercury (mmHg). The first (higher) number measures the systolic pressure. This is the maximum pressure exerted against the arterial walls while the heart is beating. The second (lower) number records the diastolic pressure, the pressure between heart beats, when the heart is resting. The results are then recorded as systolic/diastolic pressure (120/80 mmHg, for example). Blood pressure is considered high in adults if it is consistently a reading of 140 mmHg systolic and/or 90 mmHg diastolic or higher.

To accurately determine your blood pressure, an average of two or more readings should be taken on two or more separate occasions. If your blood pressure is generally pretty good and suddenly registers high, don't be alarmed. Anxiety and other strong emotions, physical exertion, drinking a large amount of coffee, or digesting a recently consumed meal can temporarily elevate normal blood pressure with no lasting effects. If, after several readings, your doctor is convinced you do indeed have high blood pressure, follow his or her advice. The risk of stroke, heart attack, and kidney disease increases when high blood pressure is in the mild to severe range.

Treatment and Care

The amazing part is, blood pressure is one of the easiest health problems to control. Here's a multi-point plan to control high blood pressure:

- ☐ If you're overweight, lose weight.
- ☐ Don't smoke.
- ☐ Limit alcohol to two drinks or less a day.
- ☐ Reduce your salt intake. (This is helpful for many people). Use salt substitutes if your physician says it's okay.
- ☐ Get regular exercise at least three times a week.
- ☐ Learn to handle stress by practicing relaxation techniques and rethinking stressful situations.
- ☐ Take any prescribed blood pressure medicine as directed. Don't skip your pills because you feel fine or because you don't like the side effects. Tell your doctor if you have any side effects of the medicine such as dizziness, faintness, skin rash, or even a dry cough in the absence of a cold.
- ☐ Another medicine can be prescribed.
- ☐ Talk to your physician or pharmacist before you take antihistamines and decongestants. An ingredient in some of these can raise your blood pressure.
- ☐ Don't eat black licorice.

Osteoporosis

Osteoporosis is a major health problem for more than 25 million Americans. Persons with osteoporosis suffer from a loss in bone mass and bone strength. Their bones become weak and brittle which makes them more prone to fracture. Any bone can be affected by osteoporosis, but the hips, wrists, and spine are the most common sites. Peak bone mass is reached between the ages of 25 and 35 years. After 35, everyone's bones lose density.

The actual causes of osteoporosis are unknown. Certain risk factors, however, increase the likelihood of developing osteoporosis.

Osteoporosis, continued

Women are four times more likely to develop osteoporosis than men. The reasons are as follows:

- Their bones are generally thinner and lighter.
- They live longer than men.
- They have rapid bone loss at menopause due to a sharp decline of estrogen. (The risk also increases for women who experience menopause before age 45 naturally or as a result of surgery which removes the ovaries, and for women who experience a lack of or irregular menstrual flow).

Risk factors for women and men are:

- Having a thin, small framed body.
- Race - Caucasians and Asians are at a higher risk than African Americans.
- Having red or blond hair or freckles may also increase the risk.
- Lack of physical activity especially activities such as walking, running, tennis, and other weight-bearing exercises.
- Lack of calcium - adequate calcium intake throughout life helps to insure that calcium deficiency does not contribute to a weakening of bone mass.
- Heredity - the risk increases if there is a history of osteoporosis and/or bone fractures in your family.
- Smoking cigarettes.
- Alcohol - regularly consuming alcoholic beverages, even as little as two to three ounces per day, may be damaging to bones. Heavy drinkers often have poor nutrition and may be more prone to fractures because of their predisposition to falls.
- Taking certain medications, such as corticosteroids (anti-inflammatory medicines used to treat a variety of conditions such as asthma, arthritis, lupus, etc.) can lead to bone tissue loss. Some anti-seizure medicines and inappropriate overuse of thyroid hormones may also increase the risk.
- Other disorders such as hyperthyroidism, hyperparathyroidism, and certain forms of bone cancer can also increase the risk.

Prevention

To prevent or slow osteoporosis, take these steps now:

- Be sure to eat a balanced diet including adequate daily intakes of calcium. The National Osteoporosis Foundation recommends 1,000 milligrams a day for adults, and 1,500 milligrams a day for women who are not on hormone replacement therapy. The Recommended Dietary Allowance (RDA) is 800 milligrams a day for adults over 24 years of age.

Other age groups should get the following RDAs:

Birth-6 months - 400 mg calcium a day.

6 months-1 year - 600 mg calcium a day.

1-10 years - 800 mg calcium a day.

11-24 years - 1200 mg calcium a day.

To get your recommended calcium:

- Choose high calcium foods daily.
  - Skim and low-fat milks, yogurts, and cheeses. *[Note: If you are lactose intolerant, you may need to use dairy products that are treated with the enzyme lactase or you can add this enzyme using over-the-counter drops or tablets.]*
  - Soft-boned fish and shellfish such as salmon, sardines or shrimp.
  - Vegetables, especially broccoli, kale or collards.
  - Beans and bean sprouts as well as tofu (soy bean curd, if processed with calcium).
  - Calcium-fortified foods such as some orange juices, apple juices, and ready to eat cereals.
  - Check with your doctor about taking calcium supplements if necessary.
- Follow a program of regular, weight-bearing exercise at least three or four times a week. Examples include walking, jogging, low-impact or non-impact aerobics.
- Do not smoke. Smoking makes osteoporosis worse and may negate the beneficial effects of estrogen replacement therapy.
- Limit alcohol consumption.

Osteoporosis, continued

☐ Check with your doctor regarding medical management to prevent further bone loss and/or osteoporosis fractures, especially if you are at a high risk for getting these. He or she may prescribe estrogen replacement therapy (ERT), if you are female. There are risks with ERT, though, so you need to check with your doctor to see how they apply to you. See next column for other medicines prescribed.

Signs and Symptoms

Osteoporosis is a "silent disease" because it can progress without any noticeable signs or symptoms. Often the first sign is when a bone fracture occurs. Symptoms include:

☐ A gradual loss of height.
☐ A rounding of the shoulders.
☐ Back pain.
☐ Stooped posture or dowager's hump.

Treatment and Care

Medical tests, such as the dual energy X-ray, absorptiometry (DEXA), can measure bone mass in various sites of the body. They are safe and painless. These tests can help doctors decide if and what kind of treatment is needed. Treatment for osteoporosis includes:

☐ Dietary measures: A balanced diet rich in calcium and calcium supplementation if necessary.
☐ Daily exercises approved by your doctor.
☐ Fall prevention strategies.
  • Use grab bars and safety mats or non-skid tape on your tub or shower.
  • Use handrails on stairways.
  • Don't stoop to pick up things. Pick things up by bending your knees and keeping your back straight.
  • Wear flat, sturdy, non-skid shoes.
  • If you use throw rugs, make sure they have non-skid backs.
  • Use a cane or walker if necessary.
  • See that halls, stairways and entrances are well lit. Use night lights in hallways, bathrooms, etc.

☐ Proper posture.
☐ Medication therapy - three medicines have been approved by the Food & Drug Administration (FDA) to treat osteoporosis. They are estrogen replacement therapy, calcitonin, and Fosamax.
☐ Surgery (such as hip replacement), if necessary.

Peptic Ulcers

Ulcers located in the stomach (gastric ulcers) and ulcers in the first section of the small intestine (duodenal ulcers), are grouped under the label "peptic ulcers". They afflict men, women and children. Bacteria called *Heliobacter pylori* may cause about 80% of peptic ulcers. Tests can be done by your doctor to find out if you have this bacteria by doing a blood test, breath test and/or a biopsy of stomach tissue during an endoscopy, a procedure that looks at your stomach and small intestine through a tube that is inserted via your mouth. If *Heliobacter pylori* bacteria are present, an antibiotic and a medicine to reduce acid should be prescribed. One study has shown that treating ulcers of this type protected nearly 90% of those affected from future ulcer attacks. Another showed that only 15% of persons with *Heliobacter pylori* treated ulcers had recurrent ulcers after two years if treated with antibiotics. About 20% of peptic ulcers may be caused by the repeated use of aspirin and other nonsteroidal anti-inflammatory drugs (NSAIDs) such as ibuprofen, ketoprofen, and naproxen sodium. Persons with a family history of ulcers tend to be at greater risk for developing an ulcer as do persons with type O blood. Certain things increase the risk of peptic ulcers in susceptible individuals:

☐ Irregular meal times and improper diet or skipping meals.
☐ Excess alcohol intake; taking medicine such as aspirin; and the use of caffeine. All of these irritate the stomach.

Signs and Symptoms

Peptic ulcers are characterized by:

- A gnawing or burning feeling just above the navel within 1-1/2 to 3 hours after eating.
- Pain that frequently awakens the person at night.
- Relief of the pain within minutes with food or antacids.
- Pain that recurs, with each cluster of attacks lasting from several days to several months.
- Pain that feels like indigestion, heartburn, or hunger.
- Nausea, or vomiting blood or material that looks like coffee grounds.
- Unintentional weight loss or loss of appetite.
- Paleness and weakness if anemia is present.

Treatment and Care

Doctors can diagnose gastric and duodenal ulcers on the basis of special breath tests, X-rays and/or endoscopy (passing a long tube through the mouth and into the stomach and small intestine).

Notify your doctor if:

- Your stools are ever bloody, black or tarry looking. (Take a specimen to your doctor's office).
- You vomit blood or material that looks like coffee grounds.
- You become unusually pale and weak.
- You have diarrhea with intolerable pain.
- You have very severe abdominal pain.

For treatment, your doctor may prescribe:

- Over-the-counter antacids, acid controllers, or acid reducers.
- An antibiotic and a medicine that blocks acid if *Heliobacter pylori* bacteria is present.
- Medicines to decrease or stop the stomach's production of hydrochloric acid.

- Surgery to cut the nerves that stimulate acid production or to remove part of the stomach. This may be needed if other treatment methods fail.

If you have an ulcer, you can soothe the pain in various ways. Some suggestions are:

- Eat smaller, lighter, more frequent meals for a couple of weeks. Big, heavy lunches and dinners can spell trouble for people with ulcers. Frequent meals tend to take the edge off pain.
- Avoid anything that will stimulate excess stomach acid. That includes coffee, tea, alcohol, and soft drinks containing caffeine. Even decaffeinated coffee should be avoided because it can cause heartburn.
- Discontinue use of aspirin and other nonsteroidal anti-inflammatory medicine, which irritate the stomach lining.
- Try antacids (with your physician's okay) on a short-term basis. (Don't try to self-medicate an ulcer. You may soothe the symptoms without treating the problem itself).
- Don't smoke. Smokers get ulcers more frequently than nonsmokers do. No one is sure why.
- Try to minimize stress in your life. Stress doesn't cause ulcers. But for some people, stress triggers the release of stomach acid, which results in ulcer flare-ups.

Pneumonia

Pneumonia is lung inflammation. It is the sixth leading cause of death in the United States. Pneumonia can develop when the lungs are infected by either bacteria, viruses, fungi, or toxins, causing inflammation. Certain people are at a greater risk for pneumonia than others. They include:

- Elderly people, because the body's ability to fight off disease diminishes with age.
- People who are hospitalized for other conditions.
- Individuals with suppressed cough reflex following a stroke.

Pneumonia, continued

- Smokers, because tobacco smoke paralyzes the tiny hairs that otherwise help to expel germ-ridden mucus from the lungs.
- People who suffer from malnutrition, alcoholism, or viral infections.
- Anyone with a recent respiratory viral infection.
- People with emphysema or chronic bronchitis.
- People with sickle cell anemia.
- Cancer patients undergoing radiation treatments or chemotherapy, both of which wear down the immune system.
- People with AIDS (acquired immune deficiency syndrome) or HIV (human immune deficiency virus).

Signs and Symptoms

Pneumonia symptoms include:

- Chest pain (may worsen when inhaling).
- Fever and chills.
- Coughing with little or no sputum or sometimes with bloody, dark yellow or rust-colored sputum.
- Difficulty in breathing, rapid breathing.
- General fatigue, headache, nausea, vomiting.
- Bluish lips and fingertips.

Treatment, Care and Prevention

Treatment for pneumonia will depend on its type (viral, bacterial or chemical, for example) and location. X-rays and sputum analysis and blood tests can help identify these. Treatment includes:

- Getting plenty of bed rest.
- Using a cool mist humidifier in the room or rooms in which you spend most of your time.
- Drinking plenty of fluids.
- Taking acetaminophen to relieve minor discomfort and reduce fever.
- Taking any medications your doctor prescribes.
- Antibiotics are used to treat bacterial pneumonia or to fight a secondary bacterial infection.
- Antiviral medications if indicated.
- Nose drops, sprays or oral decongestants to treat congestion in the upper respiratory tract.

- Cough medicines as needed, a cough suppressant for a dry, non-productive cough, an expectorant type for a mucus producing cough.
- Removing fluid from the lungs by suction, anti-inflammatory medications, and oxygen therapy may be used for chemically induced pneumonias.
- Also, vaccines against influenza and pneumonococcus (pneumonia bacteria) are available. They are recommended for persons aged 65 and older and for some persons younger than 65 who have certain medical conditions. Ask your doctor about them. (See Immunizations Schedule on page 18).

Sickle Cell Anemia

Sickle cell anemia is inherited. About 1 in 12 African Americans carries the gene for the sickle cell trait (that is, they have the ability to produce children with sickle cell anemia, but have no symptoms of the disease). If both parents carry the trait, the chance of having a child with sickle cell anemia is one out of four, or 25 percent. (About 1 in every 400 African Americans is born with sickle cell anemia.)

Red blood cells are normally round. In sickle cell anemia, the red blood cells take on a sickle shape. This makes the blood thicker and affects the red blood cell's ability to carry oxygen to the body's tissues. The disease usually doesn't become apparent until the end of the child's first year. The average life expectancy with proper medical care is now between the ages of 40 and 50.

Signs and Symptoms

A blood test can detect sickle cell anemia, but signs and symptoms include the following:

- Pain, ranging from mild to severe, in the chest, joints, back, or abdomen.
- Swollen hands and feet.
- Jaundice.
- Repeated infections, particularly pneumonia or meningitis.
- Kidney failure.

Sickle Cell Anemia, continued

- Gallstones (at an early age).
- Strokes (at an early age).

Treatment, Care and Prevention

Treatment is geared toward preventing complications. Painful episodes are treated with painkillers, fluids, and oxygen. The diet is supplemented with folate. Persons with sickle cell anemia should be vaccinated against pneumonia. *[Note: Recently, a few persons have been cured of sickle cell anemia with chemotherapy drugs and a bone marrow transplant.]*

To prevent sickle cell anemia in offspring, couples, especially African American couples, should have a blood test to determine if they are carriers for the sickle cell trait. Genetic counseling can help them decide what to do.

After conception, sickle cell anemia can be diagnosed by amniocentesis in the second trimester of pregnancy. If the fetus has sickle cell anemia, the parents may elect to terminate the pregnancy.

Strokes

Strokes, also called cerebrovascular accidents, are the third leading cause of death in the United States. A stroke can be caused by lack of blood (and therefore lack of oxygen) to the brain, usually due to either clogged arteries or a ruptured blood vessel in the brain. In either case, the end result is brain damage (and possible death). Persons who suffer from both high blood pressure and hardening of the arteries are most susceptible to having a stroke. A stroke can happen suddenly, but it often follows years of the slow buildup of fatty deposits inside the blood vessels.

Some people experience a temporary lack of blood supply to the brain, a transient ischemic attack (TIA). The symptoms mimic a stroke, (see below) but clear within 24 hours. TIAs are a warning that a real stroke may follow.

Prevention

Measures can be taken to prevent a stroke. Here's what to do to reduce the risks of a stroke:

- Control your blood pressure. Have it checked regularly and, if necessary, take medication prescribed by your physician.
- Reduce blood levels of cholesterol to below 200 milligrams per deciliter (measured by a blood test).
- Get regular exercise.
- Keep your weight down.
- Don't smoke.
- Keep blood sugar levels under control if you're diabetic.
- Use alcohol in moderation, if at all.
- Avoid taking oral contraceptive pills, if possible. (If you must use them, don't smoke).
- Learn to manage stress.
- Ask your doctor about taking aspirin (low-dose, such as a daily baby aspirin).
- Ask your doctor to evaluate you for a surgical procedure that scrapes away fatty deposits in one or both of the main arteries in the neck.

Signs and Symptoms

It's important to know the warning signals of a stroke and get immediate medical attention, to minimize the damage. To help you remember what to look out for, the initials of the signs and symptoms spell DANGER.

- Dizziness.
- Absent-mindedness, or temporary loss of memory or mental ability.
- Numbness or weakness in the face, arm, or leg.
- Garbled speech.
- Eye problems, including temporary loss of sight in one eye, or double vision.
- Recent onset of severe headaches.

Care and Treatment

Tests can be done to locate the obstruction of blood flow to the brain. The doctor may then prescribe appropriate medicines and/or surgery. When an actual stroke occurs, it is crucial to get immediate treatment. Treatment often includes:

- Medications that reduce brain tissue swelling, control blood pressure, and inhibit the normal clotting of the blood or prevent existing clots from getting bigger.
- Surgery if warranted.
- Rehabilitation as needed by speech, physical, and occupational therapists.

SECTION IV
Emergency Procedures

Introduction

This section contains information and drawings to illustrate CPR (cardiopulmonary resuscitation) and first aid for choking. Take an emergency first aid course to learn and become certified in these emergency procedures. Knowing when and how to do these procedures correctly can save a person's life. First aid for poisoning is also included.

Cardiopulmonary Resuscitation (CPR)

CPR Techniques

Early CPR is an important link in the chain of survival for a victim of sudden cardiac or respiratory arrest. CPR involves a combination of mouth-to-mouth rescue breathing (or other artificial ventilation techniques) and chest compressions. It keeps some oxygenated blood flowing to the brain and other vital organs until appropriate medical treatment can restore normal heart action.

Cardiac arrest causes the victim to lose consciousness within seconds. **If there is early access to the EMS system (Phone First! Phone Fast!), early CPR, early defibrillation, and early advanced care,** the person has a chance to survive.

CPR techniques include three basic rescue skills, the ABCs of CPR: Airway, Breathing, and Circulation.

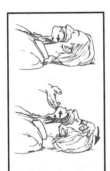

Airway - A key action for successful resuscitation is immediate opening of the airway by positioning the head properly. It is important to remember that the back of the tongue and the epiglottis are the most common causes of airway obstruction in the unconscious victim. Since the tongue, directly, and the epiglottis, indirectly, are attached to the lower jaw, tilting the head back and moving the lower jaw (chin) forward lifts the tongue and the epiglottis from the back of the throat and usually opens the airway.

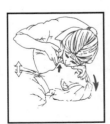

Breathing - When breathing stops, the body has only the oxygen remaining in the lungs and bloodstream. Therefore, when breathing stops, cardiac arrest and death quickly follow. Mouth-to-mouth rescue breathing is the quickest way to get oxygen into the victim's lungs.

There is more than enough oxygen in the air you breathe into the victim to supply the victim's needs.

Rescue breathing should be performed until the victim can breathe on his or her own or until trained professionals take over.

□ If the victim is unconscious and breathing and there is no evidence of trauma, you should place the victim on his or her side in the recovery position.

□ If the victim's heart is beating, you should:
 • Maintain an open airway.
 • Breathe for the victim.
If the victim's heart is not beating, you should perform rescue breathing **plus** chest compressions.

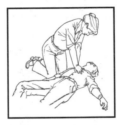

Circulation - Chest compressions can maintain some blood flow to the lungs, brain, coronary arteries, and other major organs. When chest compressions are performed, rescue breathing should also be performed.

Recovery position - If the victim resumes breathing and regains a pulse during or following resuscitation, you should place the victim in the recovery position.

Reproduced with permission.
© Basic Life Support Heartsaver Guide, 1993,
© "Cardiopulmonary Resuscitation (CPR)," 1986, 1993
Copyright American Heart Association.

To perform CPR correctly, you need some expert training. It takes just 3 hours to learn, and anyone strong enough to compress the sternum (breastbone) 1/2 inch is capable of performing CPR. Call your local chapter of the American Heart Association, Red Cross or local hospital to find out where you can learn CPR.

First Aid for Choking

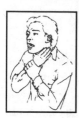

Performance Guidelines Obstructed Airway: Conscious Adult

Determine if victim is able to speak or cough. Rescuer can ask "Are you choking?" Victim may be using the "universal distress signal" of choking: Clutching the neck between thumb and index finger.

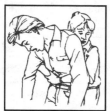

Abdominal Thrust

Perform the Heimlich maneuver until the foreign body is expelled or the victim becomes unconscious. Stand behind victim and wrap your arms around victim's waist. Press fist into abdomen with quick inward and upward thrusts.

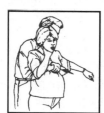

Chest Thrust

For victims who are in advanced pregnancy or who are obese: Chest thrusts: Stand behind victim and place your arms under victim's armpits to encircle the chest. Press with quick backward thrusts.

Performance Guidelines Obstructed Airway: If Victim Is or Becomes Unconscious

Activate EMS - Call 911.

Check for foreign body - Sweep deeply into mouth with hooked finger to remove foreign body.

Attempt rescue breathing - Open airway. Try to give 2 breaths. If needed, reposition the head and try again.

If airway is obstructed, perform Heimlich maneuver - Kneel astride the victim's thighs. Place the heel of one hand on the victim's abdomen, in the midline slightly above the navel and well below the tip of the xiphoid (the lowest part of the breastbone). Place the second hand on top of the first. Press into the abdomen with quick upward thrusts.

Repeat sequence until successful - Alternate these maneuvers in rapid sequence:
- Check for foreign body.
- Attempt rescue breathing.
- Perform Heimlich maneuver.

First Aid for Poisoning

Know what to do in case you or someone else is the victim of poisoning. Follow these steps:
- Remain calm and don't panic. You need to act quickly. Victims who are unconscious need immediate emergency care.
- Keep the airway open and perform artificial respiration until emergency care arrives.
- In a conscious person, call the Poison Control Center immediately. The Poison Control Center can also be contacted through the operator.
- Consultants at the Poison Control Center are available 24 hours a day.

First Aid for Poisoning, continued

Your local Poison Control Center telephone number is listed in your telephone directory under either "Emergency" numbers and/or under "Poison". Look this number up now. Record it near your telephone and on the 1st page of this book.

[Note: Many products list what to do in case of accidental poisoning. It is still best to contact a poison control center for instructions. Some product labels may be outdated and give erroneous information.]

▢ Give the poison control center as much information as you can about the poison that was swallowed, inhaled, or that came in contact with the skin. This includes the name of the product, maker, the contents if listed on the container, <u>and</u> how much was taken, if known.

▢ Follow instructions given by the poison control center. You may be told to take the victim to an emergency room and/or to induce vomiting. (This will depend on the poison taken).

If necessary, vomiting can be induced by:

▢ Giving Syrup of Ipecac and at least one cup of water. Dosage for Syrup of Ipecac: 1 Tbsp. (1/2 ounce) for children 1-3 years old; 2 Tbsp. (1 ounce) for persons 3-6 years and older, including adults. (This is available over-the-counter at drug stores). If the victim has not vomited in 25 minutes, repeat with a second dose of the Syrup of Ipecac.

▢ Tickling the back of the throat with a finger, spoon handle, pen, or other blunt object after giving water.

In general, do not induce vomiting if the victim has swallowed acids such as battery acid, bleach, or hair straighteners; alkalis such as Drano, drain cleaners, bleach, ammonia, lye, or oven cleaners; or petroleum products such as gasoline, kerosene, lighter fluid, furniture, or floor polish. These can destroy the esophagus or do damage to the lungs during vomiting. Milk or milk of magnesia is usually suggested to be given to neutralize them.

If the victim needs to be taken to an emergency room, bring the poison's container with the label intact. If possible, collect the vomitus so it can be examined.

Prevention

▢ Keep all poisonous substances (household products, medicines, plants, etc.) out of children's reach, preferably behind locked cabinets, or too high to reach, even when climbing on a chair or counter.

▢ Always read warning labels on pesticides, household cleaners, and other products that could be poisonous. Follow instructions for use and storage.

▢ Do not transfer products to other containers such as soft drink bottles, plastic jugs, etc. Keep them in their original containers.

▢ Teach children that they should never take medicine unless an adult gives it to them.

▢ Flush unused medications down the toilet and rinse the containers before discarding them.

Family Medical Records

DISEASE HISTORY

(Fill in dates for each one, if applicable)

Name	Chicken Pox	Measles/Mumps	German Measles	Whooping Cough	Meningitis	Hepatitis	Tuberculosis	Scarlet Fever	Mononucleosis	Pneumonia
1.										
2.										
3.										
4.										
5.										

HEALTH INFORMATION

Name	Blood Type	Medication Sensitivities	Allergies
1.			
2.			
3.			
4.			
5.			

HOSPITAL RECORDS

Name	Hospitalization, Surgery/Injury	Date(s)	Method of Treatment	Doctor/Hospital	Comments
1.					
2.					
3.					
4.					
5.					

Your Home Pharmacy

Listed below are medications and supplies that should be kept at home for self-care procedures.

☐ Be sure to store them in a convenient dry place, but out of children's reach.

☐ Check the expiration dates periodically and discard and replace as needed.

Item	Use
Acetaminophen ex: Tylenol	Pain relief, reduces fever
Adhesive bandages, sterile gauze, first aid tape, scissors	Minor wounds
Antacids ex: Tums, Rolaids, Mylanta	Stomach upset, heartburn
Antibiotic ointment ex: Neosporin	Minor skin infection, wounds
Anti-diarrheal medicine ex: Kaopectate, Immodium A-D	Diarrhea
Antifungal preparation ex: Tinactin	Fungal infections such as athlete's foot
Antihistamines ex: Dristan, Triaminic	Allergies, cold symptom relief
Antiseptic preparation ex: Betadine	Abrasions, cuts
Aspirin* ex: Bayer, Bufferin	Pain relief, reduces fever and swelling
Cough suppressant ex: Robitussin-DM	Dry cough without mucus
Decongestant ex: Sudafed, Dimetapp	Stuffy and runny nose, post-nasal drip, allergies
Expectorant ex: Robitussin	Cough with mucus
Eye drops and artificial tears ex: Murine	Minor eye irritations
Heating pad/hot water bottle	Minor pains, strains, menstrual cramps
Hemorrhoid preparation ex: Preparation H, Hemorid	Hemorrhoids
Humidifier, vaporizer (cool mist)	Add moisture to the air
Hydrocortisone cream ex: Cortaid	Minor skin irritations, itching and rashes
Ibuprofen (adult) ex: Advil	Pain relief, reduces fever and swelling
Ice pack/heat pack or heating pad	Minor pain and injuries
Laxatives ex: Ex-Lax, Correctol, Metamucil	Constipation
Naproxen Sodium (adult) ex: Aleve	Pain relief, reduces fever and swelling
Petroleum jelly ex: Vaseline	Chafing, diaper rash, dry skin
Rubbing alcohol	Topical antiseptic, clean thermometer
Thermometer (mercury-containing, digital, etc.)	Measure temperature
Syrup of Ipecac [Note: Call Poison Control Center first.]	To induce vomiting for some poisons
Throat anesthetic ex: Sucrets, Chloraseptic spray	Minor sore throat
Tongue depressor, flashlight	Check for redness or infection in throat
Toothache anesthetic ex: Anbesol	Toothache, teething
Tweezers	Remove splinters

* [Note: Do not give aspirin or any medication containing salicylates to anyone 19 years of age or younger, unless directed by a physician, due to its association with Reye's Syndrome, a potentially fatal condition.]

Health Hotlines

Free health information is just a phone call away. The toll-free numbers listed below cover everything from diabetes to dyslexia and Alzheimer's to AIDS. (The organizations are listed alphabetically by subject).

Most organizations staff their phones from 9:00 A.M. to 5:00 P.M. local time, Monday through Friday. Call early in the day when the telephone lines are least busy.

To find a toll-free number not listed in this directory, call the toll-free information operator at 1-800-555-1212 and explain what kind of information you're looking for.

Inclusion in this directory does not indicate endorsement of the organization by the American Institute for Preventive Medicine.

Alcohol and Drug Abuse
"Just Say No" International
2101 Webster St., Suite 1300
Oakland, CA 94612
1-800-258-2766
Assists parents, children and schools in setting up "Just Say No" clubs to prevent drug abuse.

National Cocaine Hotline
c/o Phoenix House
164 W. 74th Street
New York, New York 10023
1-800-COCAINE or
1-800-662-HELP
Answers questions, makes referrals to local programs, and offers counseling on cocaine use and other drug problems.

National Council on Alcoholism
12 W. 21st St.
New York, NY 10010
1-800-622-2255
Offers various kinds of information on alcoholism.

Children's Diseases
Cystic Fibrosis Foundation
6931 Arlington Rd.
Bethesda, MD 20814
1-800-344-4823 or
1-800-CF-FIGHT
Provides information and local physician referrals for children with cystic fibrosis.

Juvenile Diabetes Foundation International
432 Park Ave. S.
New York, NY 10016
1-800-223-1138
Provides information and answers questions about juvenile diabetes.

National Reye's Syndrome Foundation
P.O. Box 829
Bryan, OH 43506
1-800-233-7393
Distributes information to the public and the medical community on Reye's syndrome.

General Health Information
American Academy of Family Physicians
8880 Ward Pkwy.
Kansas City, MO 64114
1-800-274-2237
A national association of family doctors who govern and maintain high standards in such areas as patient and continuing education.

American Osteopathic Association
142 E. Ontario St.
Chicago, IL 60611
1-800-621-1773
Provides information on osteopathic medicine. Makes local referrals to osteopathic centers.

National Health Information Center
P.O. Box 1133
Washington, DC 20013-1133
1-800-336-4797
Provides information and referrals for consumers looking for various types of health information.

Health Problems

Acquired Immune Deficiency Syndrome (AIDS) AIDS Information Hotline
U.S. Public Health Service
American Social Health Association
P.O. Box 13827
Research Triangle Park, NC 27709
1-800-342-AIDS
1-800-344-7432 (in Spanish)
1-800-243-7889 (for hearing impaired)
Provides information on AIDS and makes local referrals for medical assistance.

Alzheimer's Disease
Alzheimer's Association
919 North Michigan Ave.,
Suite 1000
Chicago, IL 60601-1676
1-800-272-3900
Provides information to the public
and health care professionals.
Makes referrals to local chapters
and support groups.

Cancer
Cancer Information Service
(National Cancer Institute)
900 Rockville Pike
Bethesda, MD 20892
1-800-4-CANCER
Provides information on cancer to
both the public and medical
community.

Diabetes
American Diabetes Association
1660 Duke St.
Alexandria, VA 22314
1-800-232-3472
Provides health education
information, supports research,
and offers assistance in forming
diabetes support groups.

Disabilities
National Rehabilitation
Information Center
8455 Colesville Rd., Suite 935
Silver Spring, MD 20910
1-800-34-NARIC
Provides current information and
referrals for people with disabilities.

Dyslexia
Orton Dyslexia
Chester Bldg., Suite 382
8600 LaSalle Rd.
Baltimore, MD 21204-6020
1-800-ABCD-123
Provides information, supports
research, and makes referrals for
people suffering from this
learning disability.

Epilepsy
Epilepsy Foundation of America
4351 Garden City Dr., 4th Floor
Landover, MD 20785
1-800-332-1000
Provides information about
epilepsy and makes referrals to
local resources.

Headaches
National Headache Foundation
5252 N. Western Ave.
Chicago, IL 60625
1-800-843-2256
Provides information on headaches and their treatment. Also
provides physician member list
and headache clinic list.

Hearing and Speech Problems
Better Hearing Institute-
Hearing Help Line
P.O. Box 1840
Washington, DC 20013
1-800-327-9355
Offers information and help for
hearing problems and prevention
of deafness.

National Hearing Aid Helpline
20361 Middlebelt Rd.
Livonia, MI 48152
1-800-521-5247
Provides information on hearing
loss and referrals to those in need
of hearing aids. Serves both the
general public and health professionals.

Heart Disease
American Heart Association
7272 Greenville Ave.
Dallas, TX 75231-4596
1-800-242-8721
Supports research and public
education. Offers multiple
services focusing on the prevention and treatment of heart
disease.

Kidney Diseases
American Kidney Fund
6110 Executive Blvd., Suite 1010
Rockville, MD 20852
1-800-638-8299
Provides information on kidney
disease and organ donations.
Also grants financial assistance to
needy kidney patients.

Liver Diseases
American Liver Foundation
1425 Pompton Avenue
Cedar Grove, NJ 07009
1-800-223-0179
Makes referrals to local self-help
support groups and offers
educational information for
people with liver ailments. Also
publishes a newsletter for
physicians and the general public.

Lung Diseases

National Jewish Center for
Immunology and Respiratory
Medicine-Lung Line
1400 Jackson St.
Denver, CO 80206
1-800-222-LUNG
Answers questions and provides
information on respiratory
problems, including asthma,
emphysema, and chronic bronchitis.

Lupus

Lupus Foundation of America
4 Research Place, Suite 180
Rockville, MD 20850-3226
1-800-558-0121*
Provides patient education,
support groups, and public and
professional services to people
with lupus.
* Not available in Washington D.C.

Parkinson's Disease

National Parkinson Foundation
1501 N.W. 9th Ave.
Bob Hope Rd.
Miami, FL 33136
1-800-327-4545
Answers questions, furnishes
information, and makes physician
referrals for people with
Parkinson's disease.

Sickle Cell Anemia

National Association for
Sickle Cell Disease
200 Corporate Pointe
Culver, California 90230
1-800-421-8453
Prepares and distributes educational materials, trains counselors,
and conducts educational programs for the public and health
care professionals. Also supports
research and conducts diagnostic
screenings.

Visual Problems

American Council for the Blind
1155 15th Street N.W., Suite 720
Washington, DC 20005
1-800-424-8666
Provides information and
cassettes and makes referrals to
local agencies and vision care
professionals.

Prevent Blindness America
500 E. Remington Rd.
Schaumberg, IL 60173
1-800-221-3004
Sponsors research and glaucoma
screenings. Also offers educational materials, consultations,
and professional education
programs.

Hospital and Hospice Care

Hill-Burton Hospital Free or
Reduced Cost Health Care
Program
U.S. Public Health Service
Parklawn Bldg.
5600 Fishers Ln., Room 1125
Rockville, MD 20857
1-800-638-0742
1-800-492-0359 for Maryland
only
Furnishes information and
referrals to participating hospitals.

Insurance

Inspector General's Hotline
P.O. Box 17303
Baltimore, MD 21203-7303
1-800-368-5779
Handles complaints about
Medicare and Social Security
fraud, abuse, and waste.

Medical Identification

MedicAlert Foundation
International
2323 Colorado Ave.
Turlock, CA 95380
1-800-344-3226
Dispenses medical identification
bracelets or cards to individuals
who have chronic medical
conditions.

Mental Health

American Mental Health Fund
1-800-433-5959
Provides booklets on various
mental health problems.

National Mental Health Association
1021 Prince St.
Alexandria, VA 22314-2971
1-800-969-NMHA (6642)
Provides information on a variety
of mental health issues. Can also
give location of local community
mental health centers.

Nutrition

National Center for Nutrition and
Dietetics
American Dietetic Association
216 West Jackson Blvd.
Suite 800
Chicago, IL 60606
Consumer Nutrition
Information Hotline
1-800-366-1655
Provides information about
nutrition-related concerns and a
referral to a registered dietitian in
your area.

Organ Donation
The Living Bank
P.O. Box 6725
Houston, TX 77265
1-800-528-2971
Registers people who wish to donate their organs or tissues after death. Offers printed materials, and encourages public education for both health care professionals and organ donors.

Pregnancy
International Childbirth Education Association (ICEA)
P.O. Box 20048
Minneapolis, MN 55420
1-800-624-4934
Furnishes information on pregnancy related concerns through their book center.

ASPO-LAMAZE
1200 19th, N.W., Suite 300
Washington, DC 20036
1-800-368-4404
Provides information and makes local referrals for childbirth preparation classes and instruction in breathing techniques used during delivery.

Safety
National Highway Traffic Safety Administration
Auto Safety Hotline
400 70th St. S.W.
Washington, DC 20590
1-800-424-9393
Provides information on passenger safety, auto recalls, and child safety seats. Also handles consumer questions about auto safety regulations.

National Safety Council
1121 Spring Lake Drive
Itasca, Illinois 60143-3201
1-800-621-7619
Provides information on accident prevention and general safety guidelines.

U.S. Consumer Product Safety Commission
Washington, DC 20207
1-800-638-2772
Takes calls from consumers with product complaints. Also works to protect consumers from injury in and around their home caused by products, including children's toys.

Senior Citizen Health
Healthy Older People
National Health Information Center
P.O. Box 1133
Washington, DC 20013-1133
1-800-336-4797
Supplies public education materials on health promotion for older Americans.

National Council on Aging
409 Third Street, S.W.
Suite 200
Washington, DC 20024
1-800-424-9046
Provides information on aging and makes referrals to local agencies.

ElderCare Locator
(800) 677-1116
A public service of the National Association of Area Agencies on Aging. Provides access services anywhere in the country for information on local (community or state) programs, legal services, transport services, Medicaid, prescription medicine, nursing homes, Alzheimer's disease, etc.

Sports
Aerobics and Fitness Association of America
15250 Ventura Blvd., Suite 200
Sherman Oaks, CA 91403
1-800-445-5950
Answers questions about safe exercise practices and aerobic fitness programs.

Surgery
American Society of Plastic and Reconstructive Surgeons, Inc.
444 E. Algonquin Rd.
Arlington Heights, IL 60005
1-800-635-0635
Provides information on aesthetic and reconstructive surgical procedures and makes physician referrals.

Medicare Telephone Hotline
200 Independence Ave. S.W.
Washington, DC 20201
1-800-638-6833
Provides referrals to local surgeons who can provide second opinions regarding a recommended surgery.

INDEX

Index, continued

Index, continued

Index, continued

Index, continued